ANIMAL-ASSISTED THERAPY

Recent Titles in Health and Medical Issues Today

ANIMAL-ASSISTED THERAPY

Donald Altschiller

Health and Medical Issues Today

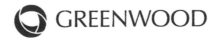

GREENWOOD

AN IMPRINT OF ABC-CLIO, LLC
Santa Barbara, California • Denver, Colorado • Oxford, England

Library of Congress Cataloging-in-Publication Data

Altschiller, Donald.
   Animal-assisted therapy / Donald Altschiller.
      p. ; cm. — (Health and medical issues today)
   Includes bibliographical references and index.
      ISBN 978–0–313–35720–6 (hard copy : alk. paper) — ISBN 978–0–313–35721–3 (ebook)
1. Animals—Therapeutic use. 2. Pets—Therapeutic use. 3. Human-animal relationships. I. Title. II. Series: Health and medical issues today.
   [DNLM: 1. Animal Assisted Therapy. 2. Program Development. WM 450.5.A6]
RM931.A65A54   2011
615.8′5158—dc22   2010046066

ISBN: 978–0–313–35720–6
EISBN: 978–0–313–35721–3

15 14 13 12   3 4 5

This book is also available on the World Wide Web as an eBook.
Visit www.abc-clio.com for details.

Greenwood
An Imprint of ABC-CLIO, LLC

ABC-CLIO, LLC
130 Cremona Drive, P.O. Box 1911
Santa Barbara, California 93116-1911

This book is printed on acid-free paper (∞)

Manufactured in the United States of America

CONTENTS

SERIES FOREWORD

Every day, the public is bombarded with information on developments in medicine and health care. Whether it is on the latest techniques in treatment or research, or on concerns over public health threats, this information directly affects the lives of people more than almost any other issue. Although there are many sources for understanding these topics—from Web sites and blogs to newspapers and magazines—students and ordinary citizens often need one resource that makes sense of the complex health and medical issues affecting their daily lives.

The *Health and Medical Issues Today* series provides just such a one-stop resource for obtaining a solid overview of the most controversial areas of health care in the twenty-first century. Each volume addresses one topic and provides a balanced summary of what is known. These volumes provide an excellent first step for students and lay people interested in understanding how health care works in our society today.

Each volume is broken into several sections to provide readers and researchers with easy access to the information they need:

- Section I provides overview chapters on background information—including chapters on such areas as the historical, scientific, medical, social, and legal issues involved—that a citizen needs to intelligently understand the topic.
- Section II provides capsule examinations of the most heated contemporary issues and debates, and analyzes in a balanced manner the viewpoints held by various advocates in the debates.
- Section III provides a selection of reference material, such as annotated primary source documents, a timeline of important events, and a

directory of organizations that serve as the best next step in learning about the topic at hand.

The *Health and Medical Issues Today* series strives to provide readers with all the information needed to begin making sense of some of the most important debates going on in the world today. The series includes volumes on such topics as stem-cell research, obesity, gene therapy, alternative medicine, organ transplantation, mental health, and more.

PREFACE AND ACKNOWLEDGMENTS

My interest in animal-assisted therapy was inspired mainly by my brief service as a volunteer working with college students who brought their dogs to a local nursing home. Watching the residents of this home—who often seemed isolated and lonely—interact with the dogs was a moving experience for me. Since I've always loved animals, I was intrigued by this special aspect of the human-animal bond. I began to read about the topic and was impressed by the large amount of literature.

As a librarian, I am always concerned with making information accessible to readers, and I noticed that there was no comprehensive bibliography on animal-assisted therapy. I decided to apply for the Carnegie-Whitney Award sponsored by the American Library Association (ALA), which provides "grants for the preparation and publication of popular or scholarly reading lists, indexes and other guides to library resources that will be useful to users of all types of libraries."

As a grateful recipient of this award, I want to thank Don Chatham, the Associate Executive Director of the Publishing Division of the ALA for his support and encouragement. The award provided me with funding to travel to the National Library of Medicine in Bethesda, Maryland, where I consulted its excellent literature collection on animal-assisted therapy. The award also enabled me to take time off from my job as a bibliographer at Boston University's Mugar Memorial Library.

After further research, I realized that the subject of animal-assisted therapy merited a reference book—which did not then exist—that would also include an extensive bibliography prepared with the help of the Carnegie-Whitney Award. I contacted several publishers and was fortunate to find Debbie Adams at Greenwood Publishing Company, now a division of ABC-CLIO, who offered me a contract. Her successor David Paige was very helpful, patient and encouraging. Finally, Mike Nobel helped me to complete the project, with the able of assistance of Erin Ryan, who located the photographs interspersed throughout the volume. I appreciate the work of all these individuals and also the other ABC-CLIO staff involved in the project whose names I regretfully don't know.

I am also grateful for the assistance of many individuals and organizations involved in animal-assisted therapy that helped me in various ways, especially by allowing me to reprint some of their literature in the documents section of this reference book. Special thanks go to Kathy Klotz of Intermountain Therapy Animals for her enthusiasm and generosity.

During my research for the book, I read many poignant stories about the profound impact of animal-assisted therapy on people of varying ages and backgrounds. The subjects of these stories include a child whose reading skills dramatically improved while reading aloud to a dog nestled on her lap; a seemingly incorrigible prisoner who trained dogs to help the hearing-impaired and whose own life was transformed as a result; and a traumatized Iraq war veteran who literally could not function without the loving attention provided by a dog attuned to his every mood.

I hope that the various stories and programs described in this book will inspire readers to get involved in some way with animal-assisted therapy. The organizations listed in the book that are actively promoting this unique aspect of the human-animal bond also deserve our support.

Finally, this project would never have been possible without the unwavering encouragement and love of my wife Ellen, to whom I dedicate this book.

Donald Altschiller
August 2010

INTRODUCTION

Among the stories about survivors of the 9/11 terrorist attack on the World Trade Center in 2001, the one of Mike Hingson evoked a particular resonance throughout the world. The 51-year-old blind sales manager was working at his desk when the hijacked plane struck the first tower.[1] Amidst the crumbling skyscraper and deadly smoke, he proceeded to walk down all 78 floors with the aid of Roselle, his three-year-old Labrador retriever guide dog. Fortunately, both survived the calamity relatively unscathed. This poignant story was quickly disseminated on the Internet and broadcast media and provided some comfort to the many people throughout the world who were devastated by this horrendous event.

Another assistance dog was also in the news some time after the 2001 tragedy. Deployed to fight in Iraq, Second Lieutenant Luis Carlos Montalvan received severe head injuries during the war and later suffered from post-traumatic stress disorder (PTSD). After he returned home, his marriage fell apart and the soldier was prescribed heavy medication for his depression. Living alone in a Brooklyn apartment, Montalvan learned about a program that provided trained dogs to veterans suffering from physical or psychological problems. He was soon paired with Tuesday, a golden retriever, who became remarkably attuned to his mood swings and served as a calming buffer whenever he felt out of control or violent. A *Wall Street Journal* reporter called Montalvan's trusted canine companion a "seeing eye dog for the mind."[2] In 2008, recently elected Senator Al Franken (D-Minn) had a serendipitous encounter in Washington with Mr. Montalvan and his loving dog, Tuesday. The new Minnesota senator was so deeply touched by this chance meeting that the first legislation he submitted to Congress was to create a pilot program to train 200 service dogs for veterans with mental and physical disabilities.

In many ways, these poignant stories—of a caring canine who helped save the life of his devoted owner and another who was able to help restore his human companion's mental stability—exemplify a remarkable aspect of the human-animal bond. Since earliest times, animals have been deeply involved in the lives of humans for food, transportation, and even companionship. Although domesticated animals, especially dogs and cats, have served as our trusted and caring companions for centuries, one of the earliest recorded cases of animal-assisted emotional bonding in modern times took place in 1792 at the York Retreat in England. William Tuke, a merchant, observed that rabbits, chickens, and other farm animals helped to "enhance the humanity of the emotionally ill." Yet the scientific basis for such an anecdotal observation was established only in the last few decades. In 1964, U.S. child psychiatrist Boris Levinson coined the term "pet therapy" to describe the therapeutic effects of dog companionship for severely withdrawn children living in a residential treatment institution.

The most frequently used term is "animal-assisted therapy," now commonly practiced in nursing homes, prisons, psychiatric facilities, and various other institutional settings. But many other terms continue to be used to describe the therapeutic use of animals, such as pet therapy, pet psychotherapy, pet-facilitated psychotherapy, four-footed therapy, pet-mediated therapy, and pet-oriented psychotherapy.[3] This popular and growing form of treatment has spawned a large number of books and articles aimed at general readers, students, pet owners, and professional health practitioners, among many others.

Nevertheless, lack of interest in and knowledge of animal-assisted therapy are still widespread. At the beginning of 2010, for example, PBS television aired "This Emotional Life," a three-part series that discussed a wide range of human social relationships, including how some individuals and their families deal with depression, anxiety, physical disability, and other troubling issues. In different segments, a couple struggles with a socially dysfunctional adopted son from Eastern Europe; a veteran of the Iraq war discusses suffering from years of PTSD; and a loving family copes with the clinical depression of their daughter. Professor Daniel Gilbert, a Harvard psychology professor who narrated the series, believes that many of these problems can be at least alleviated, if not cured, through strong and supportive bonds with others. He declares, "As scientists now know, successful relationships, more than any other factor, are the key to human happiness." The series makes no mention of animal-assisted therapy (AAT), even though relationships between humans and animals have been shown to be therapeutic. The PBS programs focus only on relationships between humans, and the much-advertised series Web site doesn't discuss AAT. To be sure, house pets appear in several segments, but they usually make only cameo appearances.

Because this omission is not explicitly addressed, one may wonder what psychologists and mental health professionals think about animal-assisted therapy as a major form of treatment and whether they are even aware of its beneficial use in certain settings. The Iraqi veteran suffering from PTSD, for instance, was shown undergoing helpful treatment solely with a psychologist. But as noted above, another U.S. war veteran afflicted with a similar trauma was greatly rehabilitated with the assistance of a live-in golden retriever.

This reference book aims to educate and inform readers about the field of animal-assisted therapy and its psychological, physiological, and sociological dimensions. Since this kind of therapy is used with many different age groups, involves many types of animals, and is practiced in a wide variety of institutional and other settings, it has been a challenge to decide on the most useful way to organize the work. After researching the topic for some time, I felt the individual narrative chapters would be most helpful to readers if arranged by age group and by institutional setting.

The first chapter surveys the history of animal-assisted therapy (AAT), its early pioneers, and current practitioners. The extensive range of therapy animals—which include dogs, cats, horses, monkeys, and dolphins—is discussed throughout the book, since they are used in a variety of institutional settings and with different age groups. Although AAT has not spawned a great amount of contentious debate, the Controversies chapter discusses some disputes concerning its long-term effects and also the methodology for assessing its usefulness. In addition, the issue of animal ethics has been raised—some animal welfare activists and social scientists have expressed concern that the therapy animals be treated humanely. To enhance the reference value of this work, an extensive bibliography provides annotated citations to selected books, journal articles, special reports, audio-visual materials, and Web sites. The bibliography also contains descriptions of, and contact information for, organizations and academic institutions devoted to animal-assisted therapy, animal welfare, service animals, and the human-animal bond. Finally, the work concludes with a Documents section including guidelines on animal-assisted therapy prescribed by accrediting organizations, a glossary of terms, legal rights of service animals in public accommodations, and several other pertinent sources to supplement the narrative text.

NOTES

1. http://www.guidedogs.com.
2. *Wall Street Journal* (2009) " 'Sit! Stay! Snuggle!': An Iraq Vet Finds His Dog Tuesday—Trained for 2 Years, Retriever Helps Mr. Montalvan Get Back on His Feet" by Yochi J. Dreazen. Jul 11, p. A1.
3. Cited in "Animal-assisted counseling in the elementary school: a literature review and practical considerations." (1995) *Elementary School Guidance and Counseling*, February, v. 29.

SECTION I

Overview

CHAPTER 1

History of Animal-Assisted Therapy

In 1961, Dr. Boris Levinson presented a paper at the American Psychological Association annual meeting about a treatment whose success he largely attributed to the intervention of a dog. Dr. Levinson, a psychoanalytically trained psychologist who taught at Yeshiva University in New York, related an "accidental discovery" about his dog, Jingles, who significantly helped a severely disturbed and uncommunicative child during some therapy sessions. The dog was left alone with the child for only a few minutes, but when Dr. Levinson returned to the room, the child was talking to the dog. He later found that many withdrawn and psychologically impaired children would also positively respond to the presence of a dog.

Some clinicians questioned his findings, and while Dr. Levinson acknowledged their critical remarks, he defended this type of therapy in many subsequent publications. But other health professionals became curious about this unique technique. A later random survey of 435 psychotherapists—about half the membership of the Clinical Division of the New York State Psychological Association—found that almost a third of the 319 respondents had used pets in their practice and more than 90 percent of these therapists found them helpful in counseling sessions.[1]

Long before the formal term "pet therapy" was first coined by Dr. Levinson, a mental asylum in England, founded in 1792 by the Society of Friends, used animals such as rabbits to offer its patients an opportunity to peacefully interact with other creatures and focus on something outside of themselves. Samuel Tuke, the grandson of the founder, described how the internal courtyards of the retreat were supplied "with a number of animals; such as rabbits, sea-gulls, hawks, and poultry. These creatures are generally very familiar with the patients; and it is believed they are not only the means of innocent pleasure; but that the intercourse with them, sometimes tends to awaken the social and benevolent feelings."[2] Almost a century later, in 1867, pets became an important part of the therapy regimen at a residential treatment center for epileptics in Bielefield, Germany. Later the facility enhanced this program to accommodate an expanding resident population afflicted with either physical or mental disabilities.[3]

In England, the British Charity Commissioners deplored the wretched conditions of inmates living in a mental asylum during the 1830s and suggested that these institutions "should be stocked with sheep, hares, a monkey, or some other domestic or social animals." The March 24/31, 1830, issue of the *Illustrated London News* later published an article noting that the women's ward at that asylum was "prettily painted, well carpeted, cheerfully lighted, and enlivened with prints and busts, with aviaries and pet animals." In the men's ward, "[T]here is the same fondness manifested for pet birds and animals, cats, canaries, squirrels, greyhounds ... [Some patients] pace the long gallery incessantly, pouring out their woes to those who listen to them, or, if there be none to listen, to the dogs and cats."[4]

During the nineteenth century, the famous British nurse and author Florence Nightingale strongly advocated the health benefits derived from animal companionship, and in her book, *Notes on Nursing* (1860), she observed that small pet animals can help heal the sick.[5]

The first documented use of animal-assisted therapy in the United States occurred from 1944 through 1945. The Pawling Army Air Force Convalescent Hospital (located in Dutchess County, approximately 60 miles north of New York City) treated soldiers suffering from either battle injuries or psychological trauma. In this rural setting, the patients interacted with farm animals including horses, chickens and cows. But there was no scientific data collected to assess the impact these animals had on the recuperating veterans when the program ceased at the end of World War II. In Norway, a rehabilitation center for the disabled, established in 1966 by a blind musician, involved patients engaging in many activities with horses and dogs. But as with the Pawling Hospital, no data was collected to evaluate the treatment scientifically.

Dr. Levinson's 1961 conference paper published in the journal *Mental Hygiene*, inaugurated the scientific study of these therapeutic activities— later termed "animal-assisted therapy."[6] Levinson, also later published additional findings in two books: *Pet-Oriented Child Psychotherapy* and *Pets and Human Development*. He found that the unconditional acceptance and love provided by pets offer a secure and warm environment for children and other patients, increasing their ability to adapt better psychologically to other people. In all these works, he described the therapeutic use of animals in a variety of institutional settings: residential treatment centers for emotionally disturbed children and training schools for the blind, deaf, and physically disabled. Dr. Levinson believed that pets serve as "transitional objects," allowing the child to relate first to the animal, then the therapist, and eventually to other individuals.

In 1977, Dr. Levinson's research and writings inspired Samuel and Elizabeth Corson, a husband and wife team of psychologists, to implement an animal-assisted therapy program in a psychiatric unit run by Ohio State University. Some disturbed adolescents were selected in a pilot study aimed at learning about the effect, if any, that dogs and a few cats might have on them. Each patient chose an animal and they interacted during many sessions, which were videotaped. The patients in this study had failed earlier to respond to any traditional type of psychotherapy—individual or group, occupational, drug, or recreational. The results were striking: 47 of the 50 participants showed marked improvement and many were able to leave the hospital. Only three patients failed to respond, while all the others appeared much happier. The Corsons quantitatively documented their successful results, which led other researchers to devise additional studies.

In 1975, David Lee, a psychiatric social worker at the Lima State Hospital for the Criminally Insane in Lima, Ohio, brought parakeets and tropical fish to his patients, who were charged with their care. The results were encouraging: a dramatic decrease in violence both in patient-to-patient and patient-to-staff interactions and also a strong improvement in both resident and staff morale.[7]

Since this research, which was performed in the 1970s, numerous subsequent studies have shown that animals have improved our morale, lessened our stress and generally increased the quality of life for their two-legged companions. According to some mental health professionals, the evidence is "overwhelming, and study after study supports the findings that animals, especially dogs, make us happier, healthier and more sociable."[8]

The growing number of these studies soon led to a more professional development of the field. In 1977, the Delta Foundation was formed in Portland, Oregon, to further the study of the human-animal bond (known in the literature as HAB). The name of the foundation refers to the Greek letter "*delta*," which in the upper-case form is a triangular-shaped symbol and was used by the foundation to refer to the triad of pet owner, animal, and health care provider. The founder, Michael McCulloch, was a physician, and the first president, Leo K. Bustad, a veterinarian. During the first international conference on the human-animal bond, held at the University of Pennsylvania in 1981, Dr. McCulloch declared: "If pet therapy offers hope for relief of human suffering, it is our professional obligation to explore every available avenue for its use."[9]

The organization, later known as the Delta Society, became the pioneering group sponsoring scientific studies of the physiological, psychological, and social effects of animals on human beings. In 1996, the Delta

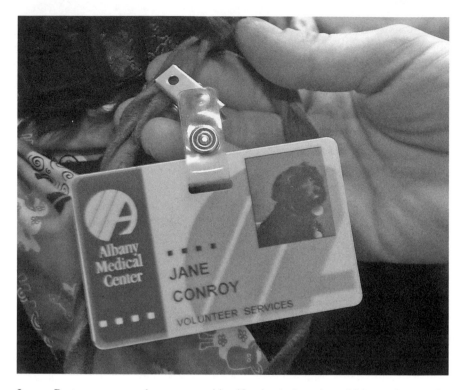

Jane, a Portuguese water dog, wears an identification badge when visiting patients at the Albany (New York) Medical Center. (AP Photo/Tim Roske)

Society published the first *Handbook for Animal-Assisted Activities and Animal-Assisted Therapy.*

Veterinarians also played a major role in the growing public awareness of the human-animal bond. In 1972, the Canadian Veterinary Medical Association sponsored a major conference on pets in society. A similar conference was later held in London in 1974. A subsequent Human-Companion Animal Bond meeting, also held in London, popularized the term HAB. Veterinary schools at the University of Minnesota, Texas A&M, University of Pennsylvania, and Washington State University also began to introduce courses on people-pet interactions and relations.[10]

Animal-assisted therapy has indeed become a respected and important field. When Dr. Levinson first began speaking at conferences about this unique therapy, he was subjected to snide remarks about sharing his speaking fee with his dog. Almost 50 years later, many mental health professionals acknowledge the enormous benefits of this therapeutic practice.

NOTES

1. Levinson (1997), *Pet-Oriented Child Psychotherapy*, xi.
2. Fine (2006), p. 12.
3. Katcher (1983), p. 412.

4. Allderidge, P. H. (1991), 760.
5. Nightingale (1860), 103.
6. Levinson (1997), 84.
7. Op cit., Katcher, 414.
8. Wilkes (2009), 35.
9. Cited in Wilkes, 26.
10. Hines (2003), 9.

REFERENCES

Allderidge, P. H. (1991). "A cat, surpassing in beauty, and other therapeutic animals" *Psychiatric Bulletin* 15, 760.

Fine, Aubrey H. (2006). *Handbook of Animal-Assisted Therapy*. San Diego: Academic Press.

Hines, L. M. (2003). "Historical perspectives on the human-animal bond." *American Behavioral Scientist*, 47(1), 7–15.

Katcher, A. H. and A. M. Beck (1983). *New Perspectives on our lives with companion animals*. "Animal-Facilitated Therapy: Overview and Future Direction." Philadelphia: University of Pennsylvania.

Levinson, Boris M. (1997). *Pet-Oriented Child Psychotherapy*. Springfield, IL: Charles C. Thomas.

Nightingale, Florence (1860). *Notes on Nursing: What it is, and what it is not.* New York: D. Appleton and Co.

Wilkes, Jane K. (2009). *Role of Companion Animals in Counseling and Psychology*. Springfield, IL: Charles C. Thomas.

CHAPTER 2

Programs for Children

As noted earlier, the professional use of animal-assisted therapy began with Dr. Boris Levinson who, while treating a very disturbed child, noticed the salubrious effect that his dog, Jingles, had on the boy's behavior. The growing role of companion animals in therapy partially corresponds to the exponential growth of pets in U.S. homes. While a majority of American households has either a dog or cat (an estimated 63% in 2007–2008, according to the National Pet Owners Survey), the percentage is reportedly much greater for families with children. Indeed, many parents have adopted pets specifically for the qualities they nurture in their children: love, companionship, compassion, self-esteem, and a sense of responsibility. Our culture also helps enhance the natural bond between children and animals, because the all-pervasive media—movies, television, books, and cartoons— are often filled with images of friendly animals.

Besides the cultural component, psychologists have long noted the unconscious and conscious psychological effects of these children-animal relationships. Sigmund Freud has written about the prevalence of animal dreams among children, while modern therapists treating young patients often successfully use animals and puppets during counseling. Recently, there has been a growth in the types of animal therapy provided for young people. Depending on whether the problems are psychological or physical, different types of animals are suitable to work with children and others. While the following sections predominantly survey therapies for children, other age groups are occasionally discussed.

ANIMAL-FACILITATED COUNSELING

Before Dr. Levinson's pioneering 1964 study, the prominent psychologist Carl Rogers provided anecdotal evidence that the presence of an animal may be helpful in an innovative treatment known as "child-centered therapy," a form of "client-centered therapy" that he first formulated.

Following up on the work of these two psychologists, several Colorado State University researchers conducted case studies of two emotionally disturbed 11- and 12-year-old boys. For three months, the boys participated in weekly therapy sessions that focused on teaching them how to command a dog to listen and obey instructions. Using a variety of psychological measures, the researchers found that these sessions provided much improvement in both boys, including a better sense of self-esteem resulting from their ability to interact with the animals. The authors of this study concluded that this evidence may support the use of this therapy for children with emotional disorders.[1]

Many therapists have claimed that AAT (animal-assisted therapy) provides an opportunity for children to experience success in and better adaptation to their environment. These children, some psychologists observe, become "active participants in their own therapy" and thus become more self-reliant and comfortable with themselves. In many cases throughout the country, therapy animals have helped children and young people deal with emotional scars. Cindy Ehlers of Eugene, Oregon, took her husky dog, Bear, to visit with students who were traumatized by a terrible school tragedy: the May 1998 shootings at Thurston High School in Springfield, Oregon, that killed 4 and injured 25 people. Mental health counselors were immensely relieved that the presence of the dog had a calming and therapeutic effect on students who became withdrawn or were not able to respond to more traditional counseling methods. In the small community of DeSoto, Texas, Tracy Roberts brought her two Australian sheep dogs to school to act as teacher's aides in the fourth- and fifth-grade classes at the local school, where these canines helped comfort students and alleviate stress created in their school and home environments. Dena Carselowey and her Labrador retriever, Buggs, were "co-therapists" at the Minneha Core Knowledge Magnet Elementary School in Wichita, Kansas. The dog provided "unconditional acceptance the moment the student entered the classroom or the counselor's office." Often in school settings the students will come to see and pet the dog and then feel more at ease to talk to the counselor. Students who are embarrassed about seeing a counselor have often used the dog as an excuse for a visit. These animals therefore enable the counselor to interact with many more students than would normally be the case.[2] Another study observed that institutionalized adolescents who provided care for a rabbit exhibited less aggressive behavior than their peers.[3] Several scientific studies have noted the positive health effects of animals on distraught children. A 1997 study published in the *Journal of Pediatric Nursing* demonstrated that children accompanied by a dog exhibit greater reductions in both elevated blood pressure and heart rates during a physical examination than those without a companion animal.[4]

READING-ALOUD PROGRAMS

The number of children who have reading disorders has substantially grown in recent years. Many educators and psychologists have speculated about the causes of this disturbing trend and have promoted a variety of programs to improve reading skills.

In 1999, Intermountain Therapy Animals, a nonprofit organization, launched R.E.A.D. (Reading Education Assistance Dogs), which was the first comprehensive literacy program involving children reading to dogs. The purpose of the program is to encourage youngsters with reading problems to overcome their fears by pairing the child with a trained canine companion. The child reads aloud to the dog, whose nonjudgmental presence

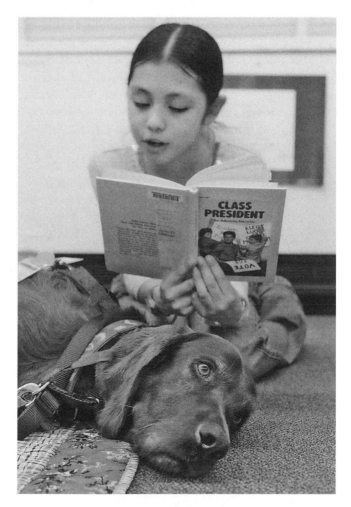

Martha Leonzo, a fifth-grader at the Grove Elementary School in Gaithersburg, Maryland, is helped with her reading difficulties when in the company of an Irish setter. (AP Photo/ Manuel Balce Ceneta)

helps improve vital reading skills. In 2000, this organization piloted an early program at an elementary school in Salt Lake City, Utah. The staff soon observed the following results: rapid increase in reading comprehension and skills (as much as two to four grade levels); demonstrated greater confidence and self-esteem in their relationships with classmates; demonstrated improved hygiene; and strong, empathetic relationships with the animals.

Ten years after it was founded, R.E.A.D. has become a popular program in dozens of cities throughout the country. A partial list of R.E.A.D. programs throughout the United States can be found at http://www.therapyanimals.org/ Find-Local-READ-Programs-and-Regional Workshops.html.

The value of reading-aloud programs has also been documented in medical studies. A 1984 article published in *Public Health Reports* indicated that when children read aloud—even though in this study no dogs were present—there is a positive effect on their cardiovascular systems.[5]

Maria S. Kaymen, a volunteer humane educator at the Marin Humane Society in northern California, joined a program called "Share a Book," where students read to dogs as part of a program to assist them with reading disorders. Before she started the program, Ms. Kaymen expected the children to spend more time playing with the animals than reading to them. But she soon found the opposite to be true:

> I found that students were more engaged, focused and alert while reading to the dogs than they were at other times. Both teachers were also surprised about how the children were reading more books during each session as a result of the program. One teacher joked that because the program is so popular, more children at the school were going to have 'reading difficulties' just so they could come to read to the dogs.

From her involvement in the program and research, Ms. Kaymen concluded that "animal-assisted therapy (AAT) motivates struggling readers and consequently increases reading achievement. . . . because AAT has been shown to reduce anxiety, I believe that students working directly with dogs might be less anxious about reading aloud."[6]

At the Alderman Elementary School in Wilmington, North Carolina, Robin Briggs Newlin created a program to help 15 second-grade students who were experiencing reading problems. Each student was paired with a dog specially trained by Carolina Canines for Services, and for 20 minutes once a week, the child would read to the animal. This innovative program improved the reading skills of most participants by two grade levels during the course of the school year. It was so successful that other North Carolina schools soon began to adopt this *Paws for Reading* program.[7]

PROGRAMS FOR AUTISM

In the past several years, some memoirs and several studies have documented the positive effects that animal companionship and animal-assisted therapy have on autistic children. In *A Friend Like Henry*, Nuala

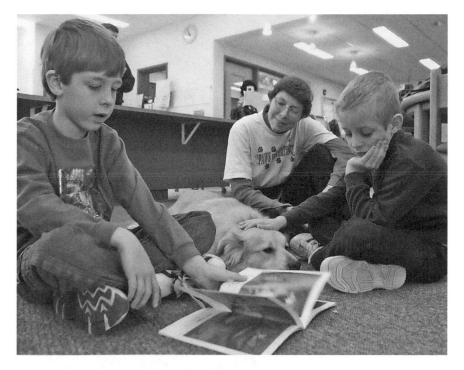

Buster, a golden retriever mix, participates in the Paws With Patience program in Perkasie, Pennsylvania which brings therapy dogs to school children with reading problems. (AP Photo/Douglas Bovitt)

Gardner writes poignantly about the profound transformation her severely autistic son underwent after she and her husband adopted Henry, a golden retriever puppy. Originally published in Great Britain and later in the United States and Germany, this Scottish memoir has received exuberant praise from parents with autistic children.[8]

Located in Storrs, Connecticut, the North Star Foundation serves as a major placement center for children with autism, taking a "holistic, relationship-based approach" to working children and their families. Since the training and care of suitable dogs is crucial in the successful treatment of autistic children, the Foundation has created a well-organized and systematic program to strengthen the powerful bond between canine and child. The Foundation was started in 2000 by Patty Dobbs Gross, who has an autistic son, Danny. After she and her husband adopted Madison, a golden retriever, the dog immediately bonded with her spouse instead of the child because the puppy was at first raised by an adult male. As a result, Dobbs realized the importance of developing a strong initial bond between canine and child and helped establish programs to breed, social- ize, and train service dogs in a variety of nontraditional ways. To provide both personal and professional advice to families with autistic children, she wrote and edited the anthology *Golden Bridge*, which serves as both a manual and handbook leavened with much inspirational material.[9]

Other scientific and psychological studies of children with emotional problems confirm that animal-assisted therapy can be a very helpful treatment for autism. In a 1989 study, researchers concluded that "a dog, when used as a component in therapy, can have a strong impact on the behavior" of autistic children who will eventually display fewer autistic behaviors such as humming, twirling objects, or jumping.[10]

Dr. Temple Grandin, the well-known author and animal scientist who suffers from autism, observed that many autistic individuals are visually oriented, not word-oriented. Similarly, dogs remember sights, sounds, and smells and thus, Grandin contends, can relate more easily to people who have strongly developed sensual traits.

HIPPOTHERAPY

Autistic children have also benefited from hippotherapy, a type of multidimensional treatment that uses horses. This approach became

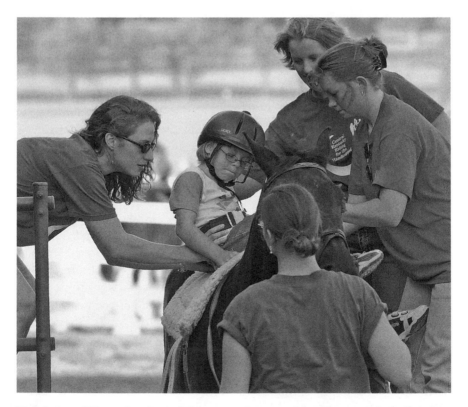

University of Kentucky physical therapy students use hippotherapy to help Courtney Marshall, a child born with cerebral palsy, mount a horse in Lexington, Kentucky. (AP Photo/Ed Reinke)

formalized after the founding of the North American Riding for the Handicapped Association (NARHA) in Middleburg, Virginia, in 1969. According to the American Hippotherapy Association, hippotherapy is a "physical, occupational or speech therapy treatment strategy that utilizes equine movement. This strategy is used as part of an integrated treatment program to achieve functional outcomes." Depending on the needs of the autistic child, he or she can receive physical or occupational therapy under the supervision of trained therapeutic riding instructors. If the problem is primarily cognitive or related to social skills development, the child will be engaged in equine-facilitated psychotherapy (EFP), otherwise known as therapeutic horsemanship. Yet the distinction between physical and occupational therapy sometimes becomes blurred when both treatments are used to help autistic children with both physical and developmental problems.[11] Although some published theses and anecdotal evidence indicate the efficacy of therapeutic riding for autistic individuals, more scientific study is required.[12]

NARHA, based in Denver, is a thriving organization, offering equine-assisted activity and therapy (EAAT) programs in the United States and Canada through its almost 800 member centers. Approximately, 42,000 individuals with special needs have benefited from activities that include therapeutic riding, hippotherapy, EFP, and other horse-related therapies. The association has strict accreditation standards and offers certificates for qualified instructors.

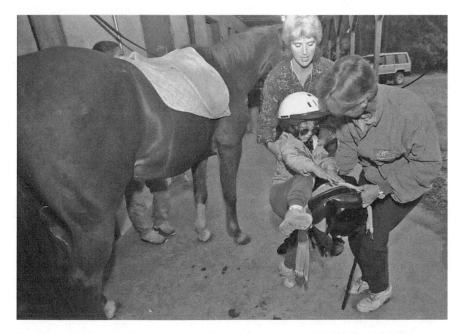

Ginger, a visually-impaired eight-year old, participates in the therapeutic riding program at St. Andrews Presbyterian College in Laurinburg, North Carolina. (AP Photo/Karen Tam)

Founded in 1996 as a section of NARHA, the Equine Facilitated Mental Health Association (EFMHA) provides EFP for people with psychological or mental health needs, including individuals with anxiety, depression, and autism. As a professional organization, EFMHA helps certify mental health professionals who engage in this form of therapy.

Veterans returning from Iraq and Afghanistan, for example, have been involved in a therapeutic riding program at the Fort Myer Army Base in Arlington, Virginia. Most poignantly, these combat veterans, some of whom have become amputees, are trained on horses that have been used for military funerals at Arlington National Cemetery. In an interview on the television show *Good Morning America*, Army Specialist Natasha McKinnon, who lost a leg in Iraq, cheerfully noted, "When I get up on the horse, I feel like I have two legs. I don't think about the injury, I feel that I can do what I normally do. I think good thoughts, you know, like I'm free."[13]

Although many people have seen or heard about guide dogs for the blind, miniature horses are now also used as service animals for sightless individuals. These gentle, docile—and, one might add, adorable—animals tend to have excellent vision, and their eye position allows them to see almost a 350 degree range. But probably the most important factor is the length of their lifespan: while dogs live 8–12 years, miniature horses live up to 40 years. The Guide Horse Foundation, founded in 1999, started as an experimental program to assess the ability of miniature horses to serve as assistance animals. Not easily distracted by crowds or noise, these animals were soon recognized as excellent mobility companions for the blind, especially those individuals allergic to dogs and for those wanting an animal with a longer lifespan. Guide horses are able to master more than 20 voice commands, and their handlers must pass a test demonstrating that they possess the orientation and mobility skills necessary to safely navigate with a guide animal.

Featured in *People* magazine and *Reader's Digest* and on television news segments, Petie the Pony is a hybrid miniature horse-Shetland pony that cheers up Ohio children he meets while making room visits at Akron Children's Hospital and Cleveland's Rainbow Babies and Children's Hospital. Certified through the Delta Society, Petie, who is three feet tall, is the only horse in the country allowed to visit children in a hospital and has been making these visits since 1997. Parents exultantly claim that their children smile during his visits, probably for the first time since their admission to the hospital.[14]

Dolphin-Assisted Therapy

Betsy A. Smith, a dolphin researcher, is usually credited with popularizing this type of therapy. In the 1970s, she noticed that her brother, who suffered from neurological disorders, had a very positive experience when he swam with dolphins. David Nathanson, a psychologist, published three articles in the journal *Anthrozoos* claiming that dolphin-assisted therapy (DAT) offered both short- and long-term improvements in the speech, language, and memory of children and others involved in this treatment.[15] His studies, however, were soon criticized by other scientists for methodological and other problems. Reviewing the growing literature on this topic, Merope Pavlides, an autism therapist and author, claimed that more scientific study was needed but noted that "anecdotal information suggests that the potential exists for individuals with autism to benefit from DAT."[16]

Starting in 1981, much research on dolphin therapy has been done at Dolphins Plus in Key Largo, Florida, which was one of the first centers to offer Swim-with-the-Dolphin (SWTD) programs to the public. In addition to the scientific debate about the effectiveness of this therapy, some critics have raised ethical concerns about using dolphins in swimming programs (See the "Controversies" chapter). Furthermore, unlike domesticated pets, dolphins, despite their gentleness and intelligence, are still wild creatures. A later study by David Nathanson used mechanical dolphins that could replicate real dolphin sounds and movements. Although this study was not conclusive, apparently some positive therapeutic results were recorded.

Island Dolphin Care in Key Largo offers specialized programs for children ages three and older who suffer from a wide range of disabilities. Since 1997, these Florida therapists have worked with children with developmental disorders, critical and terminal illness, or rare disorders. A five-day therapy program costs a family more than $2000.

PROGRAMS FOR CHILDREN IN INSTITUTIONS

Located on farmland in Brewster, New York, about 60 miles north of New York City, Green Chimneys, founded in 1947, is a unique residential treatment center for children with emotional and behavioral problems. Some psychologists have hailed it as "one of the strongest and most diverse therapy programs in the world, involving specific farm, animal, plant, and wildlife-assisted activities."[17]

Many of the child residents come from abusive families or other troubling backgrounds. After admission to the facility, these young people are soon placed in treatment to learn the importance of developing relationships with nature, especially with animals. The children are encouraged to touch the animals at the 160-acre farm, where the psychologists and counselors have developed a varied and sophisticated therapy program to treat the needs of the residents. All children admitted to the program undergo extensive psychological assessment. Their Web site, http://www.greenchimneys.org, provides an extensive overview of the

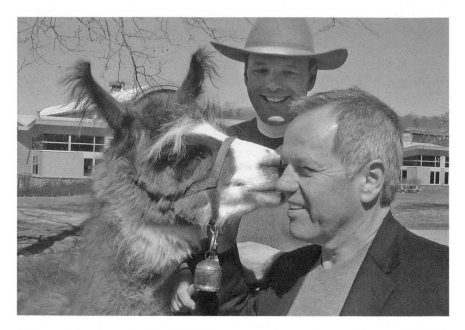

A llama from the animal-assisted therapy program at Green Chimneys Wildlife Rehabilitation Center, a residential treatment center for troubled youth. (AP Photo/Green Chimneys, Deborah M. Bernstein)

programs, along with the history and philosophy of this facility, including photographs and video links. After viewing the site, one can much better appreciate the admirable and noble work of this non-profit institution, which promotes "a philosophy of dignity and worth for all living things."

NOTES

1. Kogan, Lori R. et al. (1999) *Child & Youth Care Forum.* "The human-animal team approach for children with emotional disorders," April v. 28, no. 2, p. 105–121.

2. Chandler, Cynthia. (2001) *Animal-Assisted Therapy in Counseling and School Settings.* ERIC ED459404. (available online).

3. Cited in "Animal-assisted counseling in the elementary school: a literature review and practical considerations." (1995) *Elementary School Guidance and Counseling,* February, v. 29 (online edition).

4. Nagengast, S. L., Baun, M. M., Megel, M., and Leibowitz, M. (1997) "The effects of the presence of a companion animal on physiological arousal and behavioral distress in children during a physical examination." *Journal of Pediatric Nursing, 12*(6), 323–330.

5. Thomas, S. A., Lynch, J. J., Friedmann, E., Suginohara, M., Hall, P. S. and Peterson, C. (1984) "Blood pressure and heart rate changes in children when they read aloud in school." *Public Health Reports, 99*(1), 77–84.

6. Kaymen, Maria S. (2005) *Exploring Animal-Assisted Therapy as a Reading Intervention Strategy*. ERIC Document ED490729 (accessible on Internet), 7.

7. Newlin, Robin Briggs (2003) "Paws for Reading: an innovative program uses dogs to help kids read better." *School Library Journal*, June, p. 43.

8. Gardner, Nuala. (2008) *A friend like Henry: the remarkable true story of an autistic boy and the dog that unlocked his world*. Naperville, Illinois: Sourcebooks.

9. Gross, Patty Dobbs. (2006) *The Golden Bridge: A guide to assistance dogs for children challenged by autism or other developmental disabilities*. Purdue University Press.

10. Pavlides, M. (2008) *Animal-assisted interventions for individuals with autism*. p.75–76.

11. Ibid, p. 134.

12. Ibid, p. 135.

13. Cited in (2008) *Powerful Bond between People and Pets*. p. 125.

14. Ibid. p. 127.

15. Cited in Pavlides (2008), p. 163–169.

16. Ibid. p. 165.

17. Fine, Aubrey H. (2006) *Handbook of Animal-Assisted Therapy*. 2nd ed. p. 374.

REFERENCES

Anderson, Elizabeth P. (2008) *The Powerful Bond between People and Pets*. Westport, CT: Praeger.

Chandler, C. (2001) *Animal-assisted therapy in counseling and school setting*. ERIC ED459404 (accessible on the Internet).

Fine, Aubrey H. (2006) *Handbook on Animal-Assisted Therapy*. Amsterdam/ Boston: Elsevier/Academic Press, 2nd ed. Chapter 10.

Gardner, Nuala (2008) *A Friend like Henry: The remarkable true story of an autistic boy and the dog that unlocked his world*. Naperville, IL: Sourcebooks.

Gross, Patty Dobbs (2006) *The Golden Bridge : A Guide to Assistance Dogs for Children Challenged by Autism or Other Developmental Disabilities*. West Lafayette, IN: Purdue University Press.

Heimlich, K. (2001). Animal-assisted therapy and the severely disabled child: A quantitative study. *Journal of Rehabilitation*, 67(4), 48–54.

Jalongo, Mary Renck, Terri Astorino, and Nancy Bomboy. (2004) "Canine Visitors: the influence of therapy dogs on young children's learning and well-being in classrooms and hospitals." *Early Childhood Education Journal*, August, v. 32, no. 1, 9–16.

Jalongo, Mary Renck (2005) "What Are All These Dogs Doing at School?: Using Therapy Dogs To Promote Children's Reading Practice." *Childhood Education* 81, no. 3 (Spring): 152–158. Education Full Text, WilsonWeb (accessed November 11, 2009).

Kaymen, Maria S. (2005) *Exploring Animal-Assisted Therapy as a Reading Intervention Strategy*. ERIC Document ED490729 (accessible on Internet).

Kogan, Lori R. et al. (1999) "The human-animal team approach for children with emotional disorders: two case studies" *Child & Youth Care Forum*, April, 28 (2), pp. 105–121.

Levinson, Boris M. (1997) *Pet-Oriented Child Psychotherapy*, 2nd ed. Springfield, IL: Charles C. Thomas.

Melson, Gail (2001) *Why the Wild Things Are: Animals in the Lives of Children*. Cambridge, MA: Harvard University Press.

Nagengast, S. L., Baun, M. M., Megel, M., & Leibowitz, M. (1997). "The effects of the presence of a companion animal on physiological arousal and behavioral distress in children during a physical examination". *Journal of Pediatric Nursing,* 12(6), 323–330.

Newlin, Robin Briggs (2003) "Paws for Reading: an innovative program uses dogs to help kids read better." *School Library Journal*, June, p. 43.

Pavlides, Merope (2008) *Animal-assisted interventions for individuals with autism*. London: Jessica Kingsley.

Pitts, John L. (2005) "Why animal-assisted therapy is important for children and youth." *Exceptional Parent*, October v. 35, no. 10, pp. 38–39.

Thomas, S. A., Lynch, J. J., Friedmann, E., Suginohara, M., Hall, P. S., & Peterson, C. (1984). "Blood pressure and heart rate changes in children when they read aloud in school." *Public Health Reports,* 99(1), 77–84.

Trivedi, Lucinda and James Perl (1995) "Animal-assisted counseling in the elementary school: a literature review and practical considerations." *Elementary School Guidance and Counseling*. February v. 29, pp. 223–234.

CHAPTER 3

Programs for the Elderly

The number of Americans over the age of 65 is increasing rapidly, and some estimates indicate that this age group will constitute almost 30% of the U.S. population in the near future. This long lifespan has resulted in greater demand for social services and medical care to meet the growing needs of this age group. In addition, the aging population often suffers from greater psychological and emotional problems than younger people—the loss of spouses and family members may result in depression, loneliness, and isolation for many older individuals.

Although many individuals must resort to costly antidepressant medications, other elderly people have been able to cope with psychological stress without taking these pills. Indeed, several studies have found that the presence of animals has provided a large number of older adults with less stress and even better physical health without using medication. During the 1970s, Ohio State University psychologists Sam and Elizabeth O'Leary Corson were researching dog behavior and found that residents of a Millersburg, Ohio, and nursing home became more self-reliant and social when interacting with dogs.[1]

The following case is particularly poignant: A patient named Jed had been admitted to the Castle Nursing Home decades earlier after suffering brain damage. He was deaf and mute and often displayed antisocial behavior. His only forms of communication were grunts and mumbles. Most of the time, he sat in silence. Shortly after the Corsons brought Whiskey, a mixed breed dog, to visit Jed, he spoke his first words in 26 years: "You brought that dog." Jed was delighted and started talking to the nursing home staff about "his" dog. After all those years of silence, he began to socialize with others and even started drawing pictures of dogs.[2]

Since the need to engage in nonverbal communication often becomes an important issue for older people as their sensory skills deteriorate, some psychologists have extolled the importance of therapeutic touch. In his book, *Touching: The Human Significance of the Skin* (1971), the late anthropologist Ashley Montagu noted that the elderly derive both emotional and physical benefits from touching and feeling animals. Other studies have also described the salubrious physiological effects of touching non-human animals, including a decelerated heart rate.[3]

An extensive study of the research literature (1960–2005) on animal-assisted therapy (AAT) in residential long-term care facilities (special care units, psychiatric wards, dementia day-care programs, private homes, and nursing homes) demonstrates many other positive aspects of this therapy: the presence of a dog reduces aggression and agitation, as well as promoting social behavior in people with dementia. Although many of these studies conclude that AAT may ameliorate behavioral and psychological symptoms of dementia, however, the long-term duration of these beneficial effects has not been adequately studied.[4]

Many social scientists have done extensive research on the effects of AAT on the elderly but some popular writings have also demonstrated the importance of this therapy. In her book, *Where the trail grows faint: a year in the life of a therapy dog team*, Lynne Hugo recounts visits to a nursing home with her therapy dog, Hannah, a chocolate Labrador retriever. She describes how the dog's playfulness and joyful manner helped relax the residents and encourage their communication. As her visits increased, the author started to have a new perspective on her own life and how to best care for her aging parents.[5]

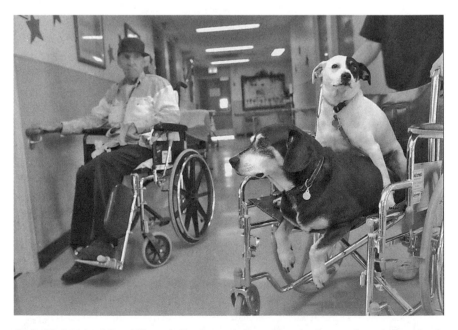

At the Neshaminy Manor Home in Doylestown, Pennsylvania, therapy dogs sit in a wheel-chair to be more accessible to the residents. (AP Photo/Dan Loh)

USE OF BIRDS, FISH, AND OTHER ANIMALS

Although dogs are the most frequently used animals in AAT for many different age groups, some older people have also benefited from contact with birds. In a 1975 five-month study of the British elderly, the researchers found that the individuals who were given budgerigars showed a marked improvement in both social interactions and also their own psychological health.[6] Several of the elderly developed strong bonds with the birds, who helped serve as a "social lubricant" in fostering the owners' relationships with other people. Another research project done in Nebraska in the 1990s found that the presence of a companion bird reduced depression in older adults residing in a rehabilitation unit.[7]

According to one study, Alzheimer's patients have shown significant improvement in their diets when aquariums have been placed in their dining rooms. Since many individuals afflicted with this condition are also too thin, the staff at this institution was very pleased that the residents who

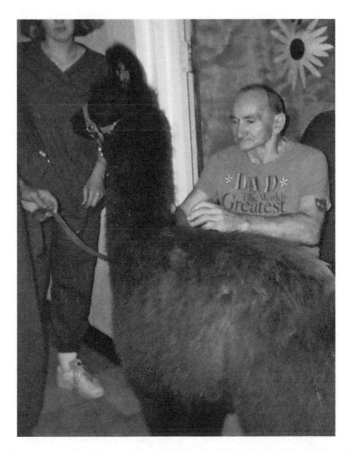

Elvira, a llama, visits Ray Bowles, a resident at the Pioneer Nursing and Rehabilitation Center in Melbourne, Arkansas. (AP Photo/The Melbourne Times, File)

became fascinated by the fish tanks were more inspired to eat and even gained weight.[8]

In most institutions serving the elderly, dogs, cats, and birds are often most suited to be involved in AAT. Whatever animals are selected, however, Dr. Leo Bustad, the late dean of the Washington State University-Pullman Veterinary School, has noted the crucial importance of matching the appropriate pet to the needs and backgrounds of the long-term residents. In a rural Washington state old-age home, a staff administrator brought gerbils "to amuse" the residents. But when these small animals were placed in the day room, the residents—who were mostly retired farmers—tried to destroy the cage so they could "stomp" these creatures, as they had done with rodents on their farms.[9]

ANIMAL-ASSISTED ACTIVITIES (AAA)

Elderly patients suffering from dementia may, in addition to animal-assisted therapy, also benefit from animal-assisted activities (AAA). Published in a journal read by clinicians who work with Alzheimer's patients, an essay by Richeson and McCullough distinguishes between AAA and AAT and focuses on how AAA can best be used in long-term care facilities.[10] As discussed elsewhere in this book, AAT is goal-directed therapy—in this case, designed to meet the specific needs of persons with dementia. AAA, however, are informal, do not have specific treatment goals, and are not modified to meet the individual needs of the client. Instead, the activity involves several residents, who do not have to be actively involved. Furthermore, the animal and handler may or may not be certified in animal therapy. Animal-assisted activities for dementia patients may include traveling to petting zoos, arranging pet visits to the institution, or holding nature and environmental programs, for example, joining a bird-watching club, visiting a butterfly garden, or maintaining an aquarium. The authors believe that this type of therapy can be effective if there is careful planning to minimize any possibly adverse effects on the psychological or physical well-being of the patients.

Some nursing professors have suggested the following AAA guidelines:

- Animals selected for visits should be easy to transport to the facility, e.g., dogs, cats, rabbits, and Vietnamese pot-bellied pigs.
- The animals should be tested and certified by national organizations such as Canine Companions for Independence, the Delta Society, etc.
- The handlers should be fully oriented to the visited institution, including the physical layout and the type of persons they will encounter. They should also be prepared to deal with any problems that may arise during the visit.[11]

ANIMAL-FRIENDLY RESIDENCES FOR THE ELDERLY

In recent years, some gerontologists have stressed the importance of "aging-in-place." This concept, also popular among health care professionals, acknowledges the strong desire of older people to live in a home-like environment, instead of a nursing home or other impersonal institution. Since many elderly are not be able to maintain their own residence, they are more likely to adapt better to an assisted-living type of facility, where housekeeping and other services are provided. Proximity to leisure and recreational activities is also important to ensure a high quality of life.

TigerPlace, a facility that combines these features, can serve as a model for this type of residence. In this 32-apartment complex in Missouri, the elderly residents are encouraged to participate in a wide range of activities, lectures, and concerts held at the nearby University of Missouri-Columbia campus. It is also a "pet-inclusive, pet-encouraging facility" based on the tenet that human-pet interaction "provides visual, auditory, olfactory and tactile stimulation and that this interaction may stimulate well-being through chemical processes."[12] One researcher found that in response to a quiet petting interaction with a dog, individuals have significant improvements in their brain processes. The architects and engineers of the TigerPlace facility fully understood that live-in pets are beneficial for older adults and designed and constructed the building accordingly. Especially noteworthy is the installation of an in-house veterinary clinic, specifically built to provide care for the animal companions of the residents. Each apartment has a screened porch and large windowsills to accommodate various pet requirements.

The construction of TigerPlace fostered the TigerPlace Pet Initiative (TiPPI), a collaborative project between the nursing and veterinary schools at the University of Missouri-Columbia. Some of its goals include:

- Veterinary care. This project provides not only excellent care for the residents' pets but also an opportunity for veterinary students to get invaluable work experience.
- A "pet-inclusive" environment offering both admission and screening for pets; residents without pets are counseled on adoption procedures.
- Foster care and adoption of pets when their owners can no longer care for them or become deceased.

These innovative and comprehensive programs have offered "a remarkable change in the usual model of aging-in-place for both the residents and their animal companions."

ANIMAL-ASSISTED THERAPY IN THE UNITED STATES AND OTHER COUNTRIES

For many years, AAT has been popular in the United States at nursing homes and other institutions that house the elderly. In New Mexico, a service called Petable Pets brings trained and certified dogs to nursing homes in the southern part of the state. These animals are all personal pets of the handlers, and the calm and docile manner of these four-legged creatures brings much joy and comfort to the residents. Other examples of U.S. programs are cited throughout this chapter.

Outside the United States, several countries offer animal therapy programs, which have also inspired some research studies. One study done in Slovenia, a Balkan country, reported on positive benefits for nursing home residents resulting from animal visits. In Israel, the Service and Therapy Dog Center has pioneered in the training of "Alzheimer dogs." The introduction of these service dogs began when Daphna Golan-Shemesh, the director of a geriatric home, met with Yariv Ben Yosef, who founded the Service and Therapy Dog Center. They turned to a veteran dog breeder, who recommended breeding smooth collies because it is the only breed that "has just the right balance of devotion and resilience and strength of character, and that knows when to take over."[13] These special service dogs have been in great demand around the world, and the Center receives 20 requests a week from the United States alone. (Please see the "Primary Documents" section for additional information on AAT in Israel.)

In Japan, some nursing homes provide AAA from small teams of veterinarians. Japanese researchers have found positive effects of this therapy in the short term, including helpful changes in the sleep-wake rhythms of older nursing home residents. Other studies noted that older adults with dementia showed "decreased apathy after only one hour of AAT for four consecutive days."[14] A longer study lasting two years sought to find the reactions of institutionalized older Japanese adults to AAT. The researchers observed the following reactions from the residents: positive feelings toward the dogs, enhanced communication with the volunteers, and more self-confidence among the residents, who also felt relief and pleasure about changing their daily routine.[15]

IMPORTANCE OF BOTH ANIMAL AND HUMAN COMPANIONSHIP

One study of animal-assisted therapy in two long-term care institutions sought to find out which program was more successful: volunteers visiting with dogs or without them. The results show a more significant, positive change in mood for those receiving visits from volunteers with canines.[16] Dr. Boris Levinson, the preeminent figure in AAT, wrote a seminal article describing the many roles that animals can offer their human companions:

"A pet can provide, in boundless measure, love and unqualified approval. Many elderly and lonely people have discovered that pets satisfy emotional needs. They find that they can hold onto the world of reality, of cares, of human toil and sacrifice, and of intense emotional relationships by caring for an animal. Their concepts of themselves as worthwhile persons can be restored even enhanced, by the assurance that the pets they care for love them in return."[17]

As important a role as animals play in helping the elderly, however, Dr. Aaron Katcher, a prolific author on the human-animal bond, suggests that pets should be seen not as substitutes for personal contact but as supplements to human contact.[18] Indeed, the following study may provide at least some succor to those that believe two-legged creatures can also offer positive benefits to elderly individuals. A nursing faculty conducted a controlled research study where a "happy person" (a nonjudgmental, enthusiastic young adult) accompanied by a 6-year-old AAT-certified dog visited residents in a nursing home. The results: "Residents were equally likely to smile at and move closer to both visitors. Three residents liked both visits equally; one preferred the dog and one preferred the happy person. These data suggest that nonobligatory visits to nursing home residents from a 'happy person' may be as beneficial to the resident as visits from a dog."[19] It is good to know that there will always be a role for dog's best friend!

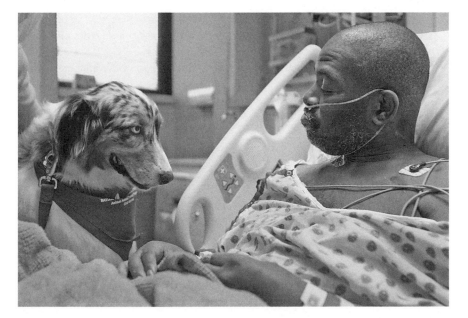

Bart, an Australian shepherd, visits Charles Denson, a patient in a cardiac unit at Baylor Hospital in Dallas, Texas. (AP Photo/Tony Gutierrez)

NOTES

1. Cusack, O. and Smith, E. (1984) *Pets and the Elderly: the therapeutic bond* (New York: Haworth), 3.

2. Beck, A. and Katcher, A. H. (1996) *Between pets and people: the importance of animal companionship* (West Lafayette, IN: Purdue University Press), 150–151.

3. Katcher, A. H. and Beck, A. (1983) *New Perspectives on our lives with companion animals* (Philadelphia: University of Pennsylvania Press), 294.

4. Filan, S. L. and Llewellyn-Jones, R. H. (2006) "Animal-assisted therapy for dementia: a review of the literature." *International Psychogeriatrics*. Dec., 18(4), 597–611.

5. Hugo, Lynn (2005) *Where the trail grows faint: a year in the life of a therapy dog team* (Lincoln, NE: University of Nebraska Press).

6. Katcher, A. H. and Beck, A. (1983) *New Perspectives on our lives with companion animals*. (Philadelphia: University of Pennsylvania Press), 295.

7. Jessen, J. et al. (1996) "Avian companionship in alleviation of depression, loneliness, and low morale of older adults in skilled rehabilitation units." *Psychological Reports* 78, 339–348.

8. Cited in Fine (2006) *Handbook of Animal-Assisted Therapy*, 291.

9. Beck (1996), 151.

10. Richeson, N. E. and McCullough, W. T. (2004) "Animal-assisted activities: sample programs." *Activities Directors' Quarterly for Alzheimer's and Other Dementia Patients*. Summer, 5. 42–48.

11. Fine (2006), 299–300.

12. Fine (2006), 292–293.

13. Golan, P. (2009) "The smooth collie shows the way" *Jerusalem Report*, May 11, 12–14.

14. Cited in Kawamura, N. et al. (2009) "Animal-assisted activity: experiences of institutionalized Japanese older adults." *Journal of Psychosocial Nursing* 47, 43.

15. Kawamura, N. et al. (2009), 41–45.

16. Lutwack-Bloom, P. et al. (2005) "Effects of Pets versus People Visits with Nursing Home Residents." *Journal of Gerontological Social Work* 44, 137–159.

17. Levinson, B. (1969) "Pets and old age." *Mental Hygiene* 53, 364–368.

18. Katcher (1983), 293.

19. Kaiser, L. et al. (2002) "A dog and a 'happy person' visit nursing home residents." *Western Journal of Nursing Research*, 24, 671–683.

CHAPTER 4

Programs in Prisons

Probably the first documented use of animals in U.S. prisons occurred during World War II at Camp Stark in New Hampshire. German prisoners of war (POW) at the camp adopted some animals living in the vicinity, including rabbits, and according to one study, they also tamed a bear cub.[1] These animals reportedly brought the prison guards, the German POW, and the local town residents into some type of harmony.

The popular 1962 movie *The Birdman of Alcatraz* brought national attention to animals in penal institutions. Burt Lancaster—who was nominated for an Academy Award for his role—portrayed a real-life prisoner, Robert Franklin Stroud, who reared and cared for canaries and became an amateur bird expert. A convicted murderer, Stroud later wrote two books on avian diseases. In fact, Stroud developed this interest in birds while incarcerated at the Leavenworth penitentiary in Kansas during the 1930s. In 1942, he was transferred to Alcatraz prison in San Francisco Bay, where prisoners were not allowed to keep animals because it was a maximum security federal prison (the movie title was a misnomer).

These anecdotal early incidents indicate that prison officials had mixed attitudes toward animals in penal institutions, and it was not until several decades later that correctional officials began to accept the use of animal therapy in prisons.

The first successful such program was initiated in Ohio at the Lima State Hospital for the Criminally Insane (later known as the Oakwood Forensic Center) in 1975. A staff social worker noted an improvement in the attitudes and behavior of some inmates who had cared for an injured bird. As a result of his observation, additional small creatures, including rabbits and aquarium fish, were brought to the ward, which housed the most isolated and clinically depressed inmates. A year-long study indicated that the inmates on the ward with pets committed less violence and required less medication than another ward without animal companions.[2]

(*HiYa Beautiful*, a video featuring animal-assisted therapy at this institution, is available from the Latham Foundation. Please check the Organizations section.)

Since the year 2000, penitentiaries in many states have instituted prison-based animal programs (PAPs). The programs involve prisoners who train assistance dogs primarily, but some inmates have also provided care for injured horses and cats. Unlike other AAT programs, the animal is not present primarily for the therapeutic benefit of an individual. According to Gennifer Furst, a criminology professor, "The programs do not have a clinical or psychological counseling component. Participants often undergo screening procedures that consider personal characteristics, such as the nature of the individual's crime and prison behavior record, but there is no regular program contact with a clinician. . . . Participants not only interact with animals, but they often work with or train the animals as well."[3] Prof. Furst does note, however, that these prison-based programs have been successful in providing inmates the opportunity to develop social relationships, possibly for the first time in their lives: "[T]he animal is viewed by participants in such a way as to influence their sense of self, and, at the same time, participants are viewed differently by both themselves and others because of the relationship with the animal."[4] One inmate defended taking food from the dining hall, despite a ban on this practice, because "I take it for my babies . . . my bird friends." In one study, the authors found that prisoners had written a "striking number of poems about the importance of animals."[5]

In 1981, the first PAP was initiated by Kathy Quinn (who later became Sister Pauline, a Dominican nun, and whose life was portrayed on a Lifetime television network movie in August, 2001) at a maximum security prison for women in Tacoma, Washington. Ms. Quinn started the program after learning about the successful AAT programs involving dogs initiated by Dr. Leo Bustad, a veterinarian and dean of the Washington State University Veterinary College. Ms. Quinn, who was a dog trainer, collaborated with Dr. Bustad to establish an 11-week educational and training program through Tacoma Community College. Besides attending classroom instruction on animal behavior, the inmates were trained in dog grooming and care. The training program used dogs rescued from the Tacoma-Pierce County Humane Society.

Prison officials were delighted with the success of this innovative program. The women inmates learned marketable skills by working with the animals and also earned college credits. Another wonderful outcome: these abandoned shelter dogs would have been euthanized, but instead their lives were spared so that they could be trained to help individuals with disabilities.

Also heartening was the profound effect of the program on the lives of these incarcerated women. Sue Miller, who was convicted of murder, trained a dog to carry books and pick up objects for a wheelchair-bound man born with birth defects. She also trained a dog named Sheba to assist a 14-year-old girl who suffered from frequent epileptic seizures. Sheba was so well trained that she could anticipate the seizures before they occurred, resulting in a marked decrease in the actual number of attacks. So successful was this program that one study indicated that 100 percent of the women who participated found employment upon release.[6]

In 1982, Dr. Bustad also helped set up a prison program of the national organization, People-Animals-Love (PAL), at the Lorton prison in Virginia. In this program, the inmates cared for stray cats, and offered hardened criminals a rare opportunity to relate compassionately to other living creatures. When one inmate was asked about the feeding of the cats, he replied, "I eat my breakfast, the cats get my lunch, and we share my dinner." The program was maintained because of the essential support and kindness of a pet food company, drug manufacturers, and caring veterinarians.

Since no such program had ever before been allowed in this prison, the authorities seemed very pleased with its impact on the inmates: participants suffered from less isolation and also manifested greatly reduced antisocial behavior. In addition, they demonstrated "considerable change in their outlook toward others and their sense of self-worth, as well as their sense of achieving a better goal in life."[7] As the inmates became more proficient in animal care, they inquired about the possibility of finding jobs in this field after their release from prison. To facilitate their employability, the prison arranged for interested individuals to attend a laboratory animal technician course. As a result, a number of released inmates were later able to work in animal-related fields.

Although many programs began in state prisons, a few U.S. government facilities also began to implement these programs. After a government attorney convinced the Federal Bureau of Prisons to drop its ban on animals in prisons, the Coleman Federal Correctional Complex in Coleman, Florida, became the first federal penitentiary to implement a dog-training program. Working with Southeastern Guide Dogs, Inc. to initially socialize the dogs, the women inmates at this minimum-security institution were trained as dog handlers. The canines later received advanced training from Southeastern and then were given to individuals with severe vision problems. After the women were released from prison, they were able to attend a vocational school and earn a veterinary technician certificate.

Two federal military prisons housing Army inmates offered prisoner programs to train service, hearing, and social therapy dogs. The organization Animals in the Military Helping Individuals (AIMHI) was established at Fort Knox, Kentucky, in 1994, and its successful program inspired a similar expanded one at Fort Leavenworth, Kansas, in 2000. Besides training these dogs to serve military veterans and family members, the prisoners received instruction on animal husbandry and welfare. These

learned skills and the animal care experience of the inmates helped advance
their vocational opportunities and ease their transition to civilian life upon
release. The programs—which greatly benefit both the prisoners and the individuals who receive the assistance animals—are also very cost-effective.
According to one estimate, the average expense of training a service dog in
the civilian world is $10,000 to $12,000, but the cost is only about $4,000
when performed in these military institutions.

Although most of these prisons house adult inmates, some juvenile
detention facilities have also become involved in these prison-animal
programs, and the young inmates have greatly benefited from them. Project
POOCH (Positive Opportunities-Obvious Change with Hounds), an early
program established in 1993 at the McLaren Juvenile Correctional Facility
in Woodburn, Oregon, taught students dog grooming and other aspects of
canine care, including obedience skills. By 1999, the Project expanded its
program to teach these adolescents how to run a boarding kennel. The
program was a huge success. A program evaluation found "marked
adolescent behavior improvements in areas of respect for authority, social
interaction, and leadership.... evidence of growth in honesty, empathy,
nurturing, social growth, understanding, confidence level, and pride in
accomplishment."[8] There was also a remarkable zero recidivism rate
among the teenagers.

Other notable programs deserve special mention. In December 1998, the
National Education for Assistance Dog Services (NEADS), a nonprofit
Massachusetts-based organization that trains dogs to assist people who are
deaf or physically disabled, was approached by a local medium-security
prison to create a service partnership. NEADS has the oldest hearing dog
program in the country and offered the first hearing dog program on
the East Coast to train service dogs for people who use wheelchairs. The
program places eight-week-old puppies with inmates who reside in
the minimum-security prison wards. A NEADS trainer visits each prison
program once a week for a two-hour class to train the inmates. The
participants learn basic puppy obedience and service dog tasks, in addition
to grooming, first aid, and canine health information. The puppies—Labrador
and golden retrievers—live with the inmates, who are chosen because they
are model prisoners. NEADS currently conducts more than a dozen prison
programs in New England and has trained more than 80 puppies, who after
training are adopted by individuals with disabilities.

The program has been a great success: prison puppies need half the
training time as dogs raised in foster homes. The program evaluators
note that the enormous amount of time and attention the inmates devote
to the puppies hasten their placement. Similar to other such prison programs, the inmates benefit enormously from their loving and caring interactions with these animals. (*Prison Pups* is a documentary film featuring
this NEADS program. Please check the Bibliography chapter.)

Another remarkably successful program has been implemented on a statewide basis: Ohio has been a pioneer in establishing dog training programs in its prisons. In 1991, then-Governor George Voinovich mandated that all state prisoners must perform community service, and animal training and care became a major component of these prison programs. An important project was Pilot Dogs, Inc. of Ohio (PDIO), which began at the Ohio Reformatory for Women in Marysville. This Columbus-based program instructed prisoners in how to train puppies. The project soon expanded to include seven other state prisons and a West Virginia facility.

Inspired by these Ohio programs, Gloria Gilbert Stoga—who had worked for New York Mayor Rudy Giuliani—founded Puppies Behind Bars, with the goal of training prison inmates to housebreak puppies that would later become guide dogs for the blind. In 1997, Ms. Stoga contacted Glenn Goord, the New York commissioner of the Department of Corrections, with her plan and received prompt approval. Nevertheless, Guiding Eyes for the Blind, a guide dog training center located in the New York suburb of Yorktown Heights, was not interested: "The initial reaction from all of the guide dog schools was: no way."[9] Convinced that prison inmates could train dogs, Ms. Stoga took five puppies that were initially rejected by a guide dog program and asked prisoners in two separate New York facilities—Bedford Correctional Facility for women and the Fishkill Correctional Facility for men—to train these canines. The inmates were so successful with their training techniques that some organizations for the blind soon began to provide qualified dogs for prisoners to raise. Prison officials were also pleased with the program. The deputy prison superintendent, Joseph Morales, noted that "the dogs have had a tremendous calming effect on the women and a tremendous humanizing effect on the prison community."

The opinions of officials at guide dog organizations were also very important in evaluating the suitability of these New York programs. Before meeting the inmates, Kent Stanley, a member of the International Federation of Guide Dog Users, was very skeptical about the program. He and his wife, Jenine, the president of the organization, are both blind and not, as Kent puts it, "bleeding heart liberal(s)." But he learned a great deal about the prison after his visits. "I realized that there are a lot of misconceptions about prisoners," he said. "There are a lot of misconceptions about blind people, too."[10]

PAPs with HORSES

Although most prison animal programs involve training and caring for dogs, some penitentiaries in the western United States have created programs where prisoners care for and train horses. These programs arose from a fortuitous set of circumstances. During the late 1980s, the U.S. government wanted to reduce the large number of wild horses and burros grazing on land in the western mountain states by lifting a 1982 moratorium prohibiting the killing of these animals. The proposed order evoked a large number of protests from animal welfare activists and the new regulation was not adopted. Nevertheless, the unresolved issue of thousands of roaming horses overgrazing on farmlands remained.

Walt Jakobowski, who ran a Bureau of Land Management (BLM) program in Colorado, learned about the work of Ron Zaidlicz, a veterinarian who helped found the National Organization for Wild American Horses (NOWAH), who was deeply involved in rescuing these wild horses. The two men soon teamed up to convince the Colorado Department of Corrections to implement a horse-training and care program at the state prisons. The horses would then be adopted either as pets by private individuals or by the U.S. Border Patrol. The prison superintendent was at first skeptical, but soon became convinced about the multiple benefits of such a program. "The deal was perfect," Mr. Jakobowski said. "The prison provides the facilities and the labor, the B.L.M. provides the horses and feed, and NOWAH provides the expertise."[11]

In 1986, the BLM and Colorado Department of Corrections formed a partnership to create the Wild Horse Inmate Program (WHIP). Select horses are trained by prison inmates, who receive both classroom instruction and on-the-job training. The participants are eligible to receive academic credits from a local college. Since the inception of the program, more than 3,000 inmates have participated. They have trained more than 5,000 animals gathered from western rangelands. Seven to 10 horses are trained every month and are then ready to be adopted.[12]

The largest BLM facility for wild horses and burros is located in Canon City, Colorado, and is one of five such facilities in the country partnered with WHIP. In addition to training the animals, inmates also feed and care for all the horses and burros at the facility. In addition, the prisoners acquire vital work experience that they can use when they are released. Originally, the program started small, with only eight inmates training 50 horses. Only one participant had had prior work experience with horses. The Colorado prison superintendent Harry B. Johnson noted that hardened criminals have become "compassionate cowpokes" because of the program. "They are proud of the horses and proud of what they can do," he asserted.

To participate in the program, a prisoner must be near the end of his prison term. Since the corrals are outside the prison area, a prisoner could easily make an escape. Yet no inmate has tried to flee from the prison.[13] "I was asked why I cared about horses when people were homeless and in so much trouble," said Dr. Zaidlicz, who trains the prisoners to care for and groom the animals, in addition to teaching animal husbandry skills. He gestured toward a group of inmates intently working with a mustang. "In a way, this answers that."

Although there have been virtually no reports of prisoners abusing the horses, a few inmates have had work accidents, resulting in broken bones and other injuries. Nevertheless, prison officials note that the prisoners still eagerly return to the program after they recover. Especially noteworthy is the low recidivism for the released inmates who worked with horses. A Colorado corrections official noted that the recurrence of criminal behavior is half the national prison rate.[14]

At the Wyoming Honor Farm Wild Horse Training Program, inmates work with their horses to provide adequate training. Since the program began in 1988, nearly 3,000 horses have been trained. Because many prisoners have never been around horses before, they have no preconceived notions about them and thus can easily be taught the proper ways to handle them. The pay that an inmate receives in the horse program starts at $35 a month; this salary helps provide much-needed money for prisoners. Most inmates that work in the horse program do it for 11 months to 2 years before they are released. According to the Wyoming Honor Farm Web site, "Supervisors have found that the wild horse program plays a big part in inmate rehabilitation. Inmates working with wild horses learn that through honesty, respect, trust, patience, and teamwork, even an animal such as the wild horse will respond in a positive way."[15]

The Wild Mustang Program, which operated from 1988 to 1992 at a New Mexico correctional facility, was established to save animals in danger of dying from starvation. It was one of the first horse prison programs to be evaluated systematically. In their journal article about the program, the authors noted a reduction in disciplinary reports for substance abusers and violent offenders. The evidence about recidivism, however, was not conclusive.[16]

Around the time the horse-training prison programs were beginning in Colorado, Wyoming, New Mexico, and other western states, a similar program was being set up in upstate New York. In 1982, the Thoroughbred Retirement Foundation (TRF) was established to find a home for retired race horses. A New York State senator, Howard Nolan, suggested the farmland at the Wallkill Correctional Facility in New York. A program was soon set up to train prisoners to care for these horses. The TRF helped develop a curriculum with the New York State Department of Education to accredit this animal husbandry program so that the inmates could get academic credits, in addition to learning valuable skills. A similar second program was opened in Baltimore, Maryland, at a facility that housed juvenile offenders. [17]

The United States has pioneered many PAPs, and many other programs have been implemented throughout the world, including in Canada, England, Scotland, Australia, and South Africa.

Although all these prison-based animal programs still need more study to gauge their effectiveness, Gennifer Furst believes that they may offer both "reliable and effective treatment." She notes that "homeless animals and prison inmates are both 'throwaway populations,' discarded by a society that cares not what happens to them (and prefers they be kept out of sight). Having inmates and animals help each other in a symbiotic relationship results in a win-win-win situation, with not only the inmate and animal benefiting but the larger community as well."[18]

NOTES

1. Strimple, E. O. (2003) "A history of prison inmate-animal interaction programs." *American Behavioral Scientist*, 47, 70.

2. Ibid., 72.

3. Furst, G. (2006) "Prison-based animal programs: A national survey." *Prison Journal* 86, 408.

4. Furst, G. (2009) "How prison-based animal programs change prisoner participants." In *Between the Species: Readings in Human Animal Relationships*, eds. Arluke, A. and Sanders, C. Boston: Pearson, 294.

5. Furst (2006), 408.

6. Fine, A. (2006) *Handbook of Animal-Assisted Therapy*, 2nd ed. Amsterdam/Boston: Elsevier/Academic Press, 274.

7. Furst (2009) statement cited on 295.

8. Fine, A. (2006), 275.

9. (1999) "Puppies behind bars" *New York Times*, Section WC (Westchester Weekly edition) August 22, p.1 Accessed online at http://www.nytimes.com/1999/08/22/nyregion/puppies-behind bars.html?pagewanted=1.

10. Ibid.

11. (1987) "Rehabilitating horses and prisoners." *New York Times*, August 26. Access online at http://www.nytimes.com/1987/08/26/us/.html?pagewanted=.

12. http://www.blm.gov/co/st/en/BLM_Programs/wild_horse_and_burro.html.

13. "These cowboys are convicts." (1987) *Time* August 31. Accessed online at http://www.time.com/time/magazine/article/0,9171,965353,00.html.

14. Patterson, Alysia (2009) "Wild mustangs teach patience to Colorado inmates who train them." *Seattle Times*, March 12 (accessed online).

15. http://www.cowboyshowcase.com/honorfarm.htm.

16. Cushing, J. L.,Williams, J. D., and Kronick. (1995) "The Wild Mustang Program: A case study in facilitated inmate therapy." *Journal of Offender Rehabilitation*, 22, 3/4 December, 95–112.

17. Strimple (2003), 76.

18. Furst (2006), 425.

Controversies

CHAPTER 5

Ethical Issues and Questions about Therapy Effectiveness

During the last century, some health-related treatments and therapies have spawned fierce controversies among their various practitioners. In the medical field, for example, licensed MDs have long questioned the medical benefits of chiropractic, osteopathy, and homeopathy. In the mental health field, psychiatrists have held dominance for many years and have occasionally disputed the professional competence of psychologists and/or social workers to counsel patients. Indeed, some psychiatric organizations have vigorously opposed insurance payments to non-MD mental health workers.

Unlike these medical and mental health fields, animal-assisted therapy (AAT) has been mostly spared from such acrimonious debates. A few factors may account for this lack of controversy. AAT is a relatively new therapy and thus has not been subjected to the type of long-term critical analysis that has been applied to the medical and psychiatric professions. AAT has also not experienced competition from alternative therapies. Since it is a nascent therapy, AAT is still generally unknown among many health and mental health professionals, who therefore have little reason to oppose its therapeutic regimen or fear its possible economic consequences to their own health-related professions.

Nevertheless, some controversies have arisen. Although most studies of AAT indicate its beneficial effects, a few psychologists and animal ethologists have raised questions about both the methodology of these studies and the lack of long-term assessment of this therapy. Probably the most contentious AAT issue has been the treatment of animals.

This chapter discusses evaluations of AAT and also concerns about the care of animals engaged in institutional visits and also focuses on one particular controversy—the treatment of dolphins involved in DAT (dolphin-assisted therapy). Finally, the chapter concludes with a list of guidelines and recommendations to help ensure the ethical treatment of AAT animals.

EVALUATION OF ANIMAL-ASSISTED THERAPY

As the previous chapters note, there is a large literature documenting the beneficial physiological and psychological effects of AAT. But since Professor Levinson's first speech to a psychology conference in 1969, there have been many skeptics about this therapy.

"The most common criticism of animal-facilitated therapy programs is that they are not goal-oriented and even when goals are identified, evaluation is unclear."[1] Some major proponents and practitioners of AAT acknowledge that the absence of long-term studies may contribute to the skepticism of many psychologists and mental health and other health care professionals, even though short-term studies demonstrate benefits. Professors Alan Beck and Aaron Katcher, two prominent animal experts, were dismayed that pet ownership had not been factored into several ongoing studies, including the decades-long Framingham Heart Study, the Health and Nutrition Examination Study, and the Systolic Hypertension in the Elderly Program pilot study. They believe that if animal companionship and/or ownership were included, the salubrious effects of this relationship could have been more conclusively proved.[2]

But even when such human-animal relations have been examined, a few journal articles have cast doubt on the reliability of AAT research that claims its effectiveness. In one detailed analysis, two social science researchers examined the methodology of human-animal interaction (HAI) studies and raised questions about the design, sample selection, and outcome measurements of the research. The authors conclude, "It is not uncommon in HAI research to read conclusions implying program effectiveness when no assessment of the efficacy of the intervention has been conducted. . . .We also see inappropriate conclusions related to the generalizability of results."[3] Proponents of AAT, however, cite a large number of qualitative studies that demonstrate the positive outcomes of this therapeutic technique. One research project even claims that every AAT study showed positive outcomes.[4]

Nevertheless, other studies note a wide variety of issues that still need to be fully examined before any conclusions about AAT's overall effectiveness can be confidently confirmed. These issues include pet visitation programs, whose usefulness for the elderly is mostly dependent on the personalities of these older individuals; one general study raised questions about whether the much-touted beneficial effects on human health and emotional well-being of the elderly will endure for the long-term.[5] In a study of pet ownership among elderly women, the authors contrasted the emotional health of married and single individuals: "When taking all the independent variables together, however, most of the variance in perceived happiness is still unexplained. . . . One needs to be cautious in attributing positive attributes to pet possession in a community setting of relatively healthy married persons."[6] The authors of this study, nonetheless, noted that their conclusions were based on a very limited number of respondents and acknowledged that much subsequent research was needed, since their work was first published in the early 1980s.

TREATMENT OF ANIMALS

Another controversy that dogs, so to speak, proponents of AAT and AAA is debate about the welfare of the animals involved in these programs. As one sociologist succinctly put it: "The prevalent perspective for AAT/ AAA research is 'what can non-human animals do for us?' [and not] what such programs may do for, or to, the animals involved."[7] Indeed, several studies note specific zoonoses—diseases in animals that can be transmitted to humans—but only devote a sentence or two in discussing the health and welfare of the animals involved in pet therapy. Although there is no "Bill of Rights" for animals, the Farm Animal Welfare Council in Great Britain issued a list in 1993 of five freedoms that animals should enjoy and how these freedoms should be facilitated:[8]

- Freedom from thirst, hunger and malnutrition-by ready access to fresh water and a diet to maintain full health and vigor.
- Freedom from discomfort-by providing an appropriate environment including shelter and a comfortable resting area.
- Freedom from pain, injury or disease-by prevention or rapid diagnosis and treatment.
- Freedom to express normal behavior-by providing sufficient space, proper facilities and company of the animal's own kind.
- Freedom from fear and distress-by ensuring conditions which avoid mental suffering.

The first four guidelines seem easy to determine, but even animal behavior experts may have trouble defining how psychological stress occurs in animals. Nevertheless, some studies demonstrate that a variety of physical behaviors may indicate such mental stress: body shaking, muscle spasms, and excess salivating are just a few of the indicators.

Although the physical and psychological well-being of the animals involved in therapeutic programs has a great bearing on their ability to successfully help their human partners, another broader issue is the ethical treatment of such animals. Since the 1975 publication of Peter Singer's seminal work, *Animal Liberation*, which outlined the philosophical and ethical requirements for our relations with the nonhuman animal world, the demand for respectful and kind treatment of animals has become a major issue in many parts of the world.

It is generally safe to assume that caregivers are genuinely concerned about the welfare of the animals, but nevertheless, many problems still arise during the implementation of these therapeutic programs. These issues vary greatly according to the institutional setting or knowledge and experience of the animal handler. For example, some nursing homes may set high temperatures for the comfort of the residents, but these warmer conditions may be unconducive to the welfare of the visiting dogs. The length of the visitation time must also be consistently monitored, lest the animals become overstressed. Serpell notes that chronic stress is possible among therapy animals, and animal handlers need to recognize the warning signs, as do the veterinarians who care for them.[9]

Some AAT practitioners recommend that visits to institutions should last only an hour, but there is considerable debate about the appropriate amount of time needed for productive visits to the institutionalized. Some observers claim that handlers were oblivious to the stress endured by the animal and noted that these handlers might enjoy the visits more than the canines.[10] There is much speculation about the "enjoyment" experienced by the animals. Needless to say, our devoted four-legged creatures are unlikely to verbalize their feelings to even the most empathetic researcher.

It is rare for institutionalized residents to become aggressive toward the animals, but this possible situation must be vigilantly monitored for. Service dogs working with individuals with physical disabilities—who help people to sit down or get up—may be in possible danger of physical injury from falling patients.[11] Some assistance dogs are particularly vulnerable to injuries from pulling a wheelchair or having a tightly wound harness attached to their frames.

Although dogs are predominantly used in institutional settings, some programs include cats, which require special treatment, such as recognition of their small size and unique personalities, during their visitation routines. Another concern is the transportation of cats to the facility. Stress must be minimized, and animal handlers need to adapt the care of these smaller animals (especially creatures that may easily hide) to the structural design of the institutions they visit. It is important to note the distinction between these domestic animals. Cats, which are famously independent, differ from dogs which often like to be near their owners or handlers.

Other animals such as parrots have been increasingly used for therapy in institutional settings, but they require much more attention, both for their physical and emotional needs. Avian specialists have noted that their specialized care necessitates sufficient lighting, special diet, good air quality, and constant interactions with people. In one unpublished study, the authors questioned whether it is indeed "ethically appropriate to place birds in these settings at all."[12]

Similarly, the use of capuchin monkeys—who assist wheelchair-bound and physically disabled individuals—has also raised serious concerns. The monkeys are occasionally neutered and some teeth are removed to avoid possible harm to humans. Serpell also notes that electric-shock collars have at times been placed on the monkeys to prevent possible aggressive behavior and the use of such harsh restraining devices raises serious ethical issues.[13]

Although it is widely believed that AAT/AAA is good for animals as well as humans, many animals do not respond well to the training or the activities involved in this therapy. "The fact that a large number of animals fail to respond to the nurturing and training they receive has not generally been taken as evidence that they do not want to, or are unable to, participate. Instead, practitioners tend to respond to failure by changing the selection or the training procedures, as if the animals are theoretically capable of responding positively to any demands made of them."[14]

Some animal behavior specialists have noted that assistance and therapy animals have "little control over their social lives and . . . cannot avoid or escape unwelcome or unpleasant social intrusions. Denying animals control over their physical and social environment is also known to have adverse effects on their physical and mental well-being."[15] Other authors have noted that "stress-related fatigue" is probably most acute for therapy animals who reside in institutions, for example, psychiatric live-in facilities, penitentiaries, and nursing homes, where the animals are "on call" all the time. Similar to humans, these animals must be offered occasional time to leave the facility to ensure both their own psychological well-being and their physical comfort.

Another perennial problem affecting therapy animals is the constant changeover of human owners and handlers, which may cause undue stress. In addition, "Many assistance animal practitioners have little firsthand knowledge of animal needs other than hygienic veterinary or training considerations . . . The organizations keeping and rearing these animals should recognize their ethical obligations by doing everything possible to minimize the distress."[16]

Animal welfare experts and many concerned dog lovers also worry about the problems of inbreeding. Since many service and assistance dogs are purebred canines (e.g., Labrador and golden retrievers, German shepherds), some experts warn that generational dog inbreeding creates a greater susceptibility to numerous physical ailments and diseases and even psychological problems. Although these dogs generally display the essential temperament and gentleness required for working with their human companions, animal biologists express concern about the long-term impact of such breeding practices.

This chapter earlier alluded to the considerable literature on zoonoses— diseases transmitted by animals to humans. But assistance and service animals are also susceptible to a wide variety of ailments that they do not transmit. It is noteworthy that a poignant and beautifully illustrated work, *Dog Heroes of September 11th: A Tribute to America's Search and Rescue Dogs*, which describes the emotional and physical support that canines provided the rescue workers and firefighters in the aftermath of that tragedy, also briefly discusses the subsequent health of these animals.[17] Understandably, many studies have examined the long-term health problems suffered by the valiant rescue workers, but there is reportedly only one major scientific study of the medical and behavioral effects that the Twin Tower collapse had on the search-and-rescue (SAR) dogs. Fortunately, there was "no evidence that responding dogs developed adverse effects related to their work."[18] The veterinarians who authored this study, however, note the importance of "continued vigilance . . . for the benefit of the SAR dogs and the human responders."

As the demand for AAT continues to grow, it is noteworthy that a formal code of ethics for the treatment of these animals has not yet been formulated. Serpell has compiled the following useful and compassionate list of preliminary recommendations and guidelines for AAT/AAA practitioners:[19]

1. Those involved in preparing or using animals for service and therapy need to educate themselves regarding the particular social and behavioral needs of these animals, both to avoid the consequences of social and behavioral deprivation and to permit animals a degree of control over the levels of social and environmental stimulation they receive.

2. AAT practitioners need to understand that close physical contact with strangers may be inherently stressful for many animals and recognize the signs of stress when they appear. Ideally, visitation and therapy sessions should be terminated before, rather than after, such symptoms are manifested.

3. In residential programs, one or more staff persons should be held primarily accountable for the care and welfare of any therapy animal and for supervising all interactions with inmates/residents. No animal should be left unsupervised in a situation where its welfare might reasonably be considered a risk.

4. Nondomestic species should not be used for AAA/T or assistance work except under exceptional circumstances (e.g., wildlife rehabilitation) and where appropriate care can be guaranteed.

5. On the basis of current evidence, so-called dolphin swim programs cannot be ethically justified. (For more information on this issue, see further below.)

6. During the process of rearing and training assistance animals, transitions between successive handlers or owners should be carried out in such a way as to cause minimal distress due to the disruption of pre-existing social bonds.

7. Efforts and resources should be dedicated to developing methods of accurately identifying and distributing suitable assistance animals from

among those relinquished to animal shelters. These efforts should include research into appropriate behavioral screening methods.

8. The present level of assistance dog "failure" is ethically unacceptable and needs to be reduced. The "industry" should be more aware of the problems inherent in the use of closed purebred populations of service and assistance dogs. The potential benefits of outcrossing to other populations and of crossbreeding should be explored to reduce the prevalence of deleterious genetic diseases, as well as improving infectious disease resistance.

9. The "industry" should give more attention to ensuring that assistance and service animals are prepared adequately during development for the tasks and roles assigned to them as adults.

10. Alternatives to the use of aversive conditioning in the training of assistance animals need to be investigated and developed wherever possible, particularly with respect to the training of wheelchair dogs. If necessary, the "industry" should consider discontinuing the use of animals for particular purposes if alternatives to aversive conditioning cannot be found.

11. More attention should be given to the design and construction of animal-friendly equipment and holding facilities for AAA/T and assistance animals.

12. Continuing education programs for animal practitioners and end users should be available to ensure that animals are handled, cared for, and used correctly.

DOLPHIN-ASSISTED THERAPY

The use of dolphins in AAT—dolphin-assisted therapy (DAT)—was discussed in an earlier chapter regarding its use with children with autism. The Web contains numerous sites extolling the virtues of the broader swimming-with-dolphin (SWD) programs, which occasionally note DAT and its beneficial effects on different types of individuals, including children with autism. It should be noted that many of these Web sites are sponsored by tourist attractions, which lure visitors by inviting them to participate in these very expensive recreational programs.

The major scientific DAT proponent is Dr. David E. Nathanson, a psychologist, who has written several articles about the positive effect of dolphins on mentally retarded and autistic children.[20] But other scientists have raised serious doubts about the effectiveness of DAT and even claim it might be harmful to the children. A study by the British Whale and Dolphin Conservation Society cited instances where agitated dolphins confined to a tank have bitten people, and may thus spread a variety of bacterial or other infections.[21] Dr. Tracy L. Humphries evaluated six studies and could not find data to support "the notion that using interactions with dolphins is any more effective than other reinforcers for improving child learning or social-emotional development."[22] Other scientists speculate that the general eagerness to believe in the healing powers of dolphins stems from a variety of cultural factors, including the popularity of the television program *Flipper* and the endearing "cuteness" of these seaborne mammals, who always seem to be smiling.

It is particularly noteworthy that Betsy A. Smith—the pioneering researcher who trumpeted the value of dolphin therapy during the 1970s— decided to suspend her work in 1992 because of her growing ethical concerns about exploiting these captive mammals.

The World Society for the Protection of Animals has also condemned SWD and other dolphin-human interaction programs, and the organization describes the following problem with these programs. In captivity, dolphins are confined to pens of about 30 feet in length but dolphins in the wild swim up to 40 miles per day, so their confinement cripples their normal routine. This small living area also prevents captive dolphins from performing echolocation—a sensory system found in bats and dolphins where high-pitched sounds are emitted and their echoes are interpreted to determine the direction and distance of objects—a crucial component for their ability to navigate waters.

The Whale and Dolphin Conservation Society (WDCS) has called for a ban on DAT. The organization's Web site notes the following problems:

- There is no scientific evidence to prove that the therapy is effective.
- There are no official standards or regulation governing the industry.
- Dolphins are removed from the wild to stock the growing number of DAT facilities, and this has both serious conservation and welfare implications for the animals.
- Both people and animals can be exposed to infection and injury when participating in DAT.

Research Autism, the only British charity exclusively dedicated to research into interventions in autism, supports the WDCS ban. Their Web site also explains their opposition: "Dolphin therapy presents a number of ethical issues, and some physical threats, to both people and dolphins, which may be difficult to overcome. Of particular concern are the potential for aggressive behaviour by dolphins towards swimmers and the potential for disease transmission. Alternatives to dolphin therapy are available, at a much lower financial cost and without the potential harm to the people and the dolphins involved."[23]

CONCLUSION

In many ways, AAT is similar to other psychological and physical therapeutic techniques: a rigorous statistical model is used to evaluate its effectiveness; a growing literature (book and journal articles) discusses its multifarious aspects; it is practiced in a wide variety of institutional and individual settings; and the popular print and electronic media often feature stories about it. Other similarities with health-related treatments are the questions raised about the methodology of some studies and the long-term beneficial effects of these treatments.

In one crucial aspect, however, AAT is very different from psychological counseling, medical and physical treatment of patients, and other health-related care giving activities. The caregivers—in this case, the animals—are voiceless. So it is incumbent upon their two-legged companions to ensure that their physical well-being and emotional health are always considered and adequately addressed.

NOTES

1. Beck, A. M. and Katcher, A. H. (2003)"Future directions in human-animal bond research." *American Behavioral Scientist*, 47, 85.

2. Ibid, p. 87.

3. Wilson, C. and Barker, S. (2003) "Challenges in designing human-animal interaction research." *American Behavioral Scientist*, 47, 25.

4. Nimer, J. and Lundahl, B. (2007), "Animal-assisted therapy: a meta-analysis." *Anthrozoos*, 20, 226.

5. Hatch, A. (2007) "The view from all fours: A look at an animal-assisted program from the animals' perspective." *Anthrozoos*, 20, 37.

6. Katcher, A. H. and Beck, A. M. (1983) "Pet possession and life satisfaction in
elderly women." *New perspectives on our lives with companion animals*. Philadelphia: University of Pennsylvania Press, 316.

7. Hatch (2007) 38.

8. Hubrecht R. and Turner, D. C. "Companion Animal Welfare in Private and Institutional Settings." In Wilson, C. C. and Turner, D. C. (1998) *Companion Animals in Human Health*, 269.

9. Serpell, J. A., Coppinger, R. and Fine, H. (2006) "Welfare considerations in therapy and assistance animals." In Fine (ed.) *Handbook on animal-assisted therapy: Theoretical foundations and guidelines for practice*, 457

10. Ibid, 460.

11. Hubrecht (1998), 273.

12. Cited in Serpell (2006), 458.

13. Ibid, 458.

14. Serpell (2006), 454.

15. Ibid, 456.

16. Ibid, 463.

17. Bauer, Nona Kilgore (2006) *Dog heroes of September 11th: A tribute to America's search and rescue dogs*. Allenhurst, NJ: Kennel Club Books.

18. Otto, C. M. et al. (2004) "Medical and behavioral surveillance of dogs deployed to the World Trade Center and the Pentagon from October 2001 to

June 2002." *Journal of the American Veterinary Medical Association (JAVMA)*. 225, September 15, 861.

   19. Serpell (2006) 469–470.

   20. Nathanson, D. E. (1998) "Long-term effectiveness of dolphin-assisted therapy for children with severe disabilities" *Anthrozoos* 11, 22–32. (Other articles were also published in *Anthrozoos*).

   21. http://mundoazul.org/habitats-species/whales-and-dolphins/freedom-for -dolphins/dolphin-therapy/.

   22. Skeptic's Dictionary (http://www.skepdic.com/dat.html).

   23. http://www.researchautism.net/autism_treatments_therapies_intervention .ikml?ra=64&infolevel=4.

SECTION III

Bibliography and Resources

Bibliography

INTRODUCTION

Since the publication of Dr. Boris Levinson's seminal work, *Pet-Oriented Child Psychotherapy*, in 1969, information on animal-assisted therapy has grown exponentially. It seems that hardly a week passes without an article appearing in a newspaper or magazine or a local or national television newscast featuring a poignant story about animals visiting hospital patients, mental institutions, nursing homes, institutionalized children, or inmates in penitentiaries, among others. Complementing the popular media coverage, academic journals have published an enormous number of scholarly studies discussing the psychological, medical, health and social benefits derived from this unique application of the human-animal bond—generally known as pet- or animal-assisted therapy.

Although a comprehensive bibliography would be impossible to compile, the following section attempts to provide a representative selection of this vast and burgeoning information. The bibliography includes books, magazine and journal articles, videos, and listings of organizations and research centers. To assemble this extensive bibliography—which includes numerous original annotations—I have scoured print indexes, electronic databases, library catalogs, bibliographies in books and journals, and the Internet. I have also divided the bibliography into discrete topical categories to assist researchers looking for specialized information. As far as I can determine, the following annotated listing of videos will be the longest and most detailed coverage currently available.

Since the literature on the topic is so vast, I have spent considerable time deciding *what not to include*. As a librarian, I have noticed that too many published bibliographies follow an "everything but the kitchen sink" approach to listing citations. Unfortunately, the resulting bibliographies often bewilder readers, who are overwhelmed by their length. I have tried to include article citations that are representative of the literature. In my annotated entries of books and videos, however, I was less selective in order to provide more information for readers to make their own selection.

I have always had professional respect for the work of the Boston University Interlibrary Loan department, and my personal appreciation has now been further enhanced by their invaluable assistance to me in obtaining hard-to-find items.

I hope that this bibliography will provide general readers, students, mental and healthcare professionals, animal care specialists, and many others with a helpful and easy-to-use reference source on this topic of growing importance. As a recipient of the Carnegie-Whitney Award sponsored by the American Library Association, I was able to make a special visit to the National Library of Medicine in Bethesda, Maryland, to do some of my research. I appreciate the financial support from this award and the assistance of Mr. Don Chatham, the associate executive director of the Publishing Division of the American Library Association.

Books

Anderson, P. Elizabeth. *The Powerful bond between people and pets: Our boundless connections to companion animals*. Westport, CT: Praeger, 2008.

Although most of this book deals with the multifaceted aspects of the human-animal bond, a chapter on animal-assisted therapy provides an excellent and informative overview of the topic.

Arkow, Phil. *Animal-assisted therapy and activities: a study resource guide and bibliography for the use of companion animals in selected therapies*. (Published by author) Phil Arkow, 37 Hillside Road, Stratford, NJ 08084, 2004, 9th ed.

Although containing many dated references, this self-published work still serves as a useful manual, basic guide, directory, and bibliography. The compiler has been involved in animal-assisted therapy for many years and teaches courses on the subject.

Arnold, Jennifer. *Through a dog's eyes*. New York: Spiegel & Grau, 2010.

Written by the founder of a service dog training school, the author discusses her techniques honed over two decades for training dogs and understanding their complex relationships with people. (See "Videos" section)

Beck, Alan M. and Aaron Katcher. *Between pets and people: the importance of animal companionship*. West Lafayette, IN: Purdue University Press, 1996.

Similar to the Anderson volume (see above), this work also explores the richness of human-animal relationships. The chapter on pets as therapists offers an interesting overview of the topic, enhanced with touching photographs of assistance animals and their human companions.

Becker, Marty. *The healing power of pets: harnessing the amazing ability of pets to make and keep people happy and healthy.* New York: Hyperion, 2002.

Written by a veterinarian who appears on television and has a syndicated newspaper column on pets, this book exudes the author's enthusiastic love of animals. The chapters on assistance animals and the benefits of equine therapy are particularly worthwhile.

Burch, Mary R. *Wanted! Animal volunteers.* New York: Howell Book House, 2003.

A general manual recommending the best type of animal (dog, cat, horse, etc.) that pet owners can use in different therapeutic and institutionalized settings. Unfortunately, the book provides no bibliographic references.

Bustad, Leo K. *Animals, aging, and the aged.* Minneapolis: University of Minnesota Press, 1980.

Written by a prominent veterinarian, this book contains revised versions of his 1979 lectures delivered at the Duluth and St. Paul campuses of the University of Minnesota.

Chandler, Cynthia K. *Animal assisted therapy in counseling.* New York: Routledge, 2005.

Written by a certified animal-assistance therapist, this book provides specific guidelines for training a pet, counseling through different techniques, and dealing with special communities (the elderly, hospices, prisons, etc.) An interesting chapter discusses human-animal relationships in South Korea.

Coudert, Jo. *The good shepherd: a special dog's gift of healing.* Kansas City, MO: Andrews McMeel, 1998.

Jeremy Davis, an Oregon teenager who died of bone cancer, was inseparable from his German shepherd, Grizzly. After Jeremy's death, his mother, Lana, helped found two organizations: the Good Shepherd Association and the Utah Animal-Assisted Therapy Association, where owners and their animal companions (including cats, a rabbit, and dogs) visit sick children in hospitals or those with disabilities, bringing them comfort and cheer.

Crawford, Jacqueline J. and Karen A. Pomerinke. *Therapy pets: the animal-human healing partnership.* Amherst, NY: Prometheus Books, 2003.

This book provides inspiring stories of individuals of all ages and in different regions of the country who have been helped through animal-assisted therapy. One section discusses the successful use of hippotherapy (therapy with horses) for both physical rehabilitation and psychological treatment.

Cusack, Odean and Elaine Smith. *Pets and the elderly: the therapeutic bond.* New York: Haworth Press, 1984.

One of the earliest works examining the profound social and psychological benefits derived by the elderly from contact with animals. The book contains many individual stories of the salubrious effects of these interactions, which are enhanced by several photographs interspersed throughout the text. This work has been cited in academic journal articles for its range of information.

David, Kathy Diamond. *Therapy dogs: training your dog to reach others.* Wenatchee, WA: Dogwise Publishing, 2002, 2nd ed.

A practical and very useful guide including specific training techniques, such as how to avoid inadvertent animal-induced injuries and the role of the handler in therapeutic settings. A section on "what to wear" offers helpful information that many pet owners may not know, for example, do not include last names on identification badges in psychiatric facilities, which patients might later use to contact the handler.

Davis, Marcie and Melissa Bunnell. *Working like dogs: the service dog guidebook.* Crawford, CO: Alpine Publications, 2007.

The authors, a woman with paraplegia, who has an assistance dog and a counselor, provide a wide range of information for potential service dog applicants, including travel information, training, daily care, grooming, puppy raising, and retirement of the animal, among many other topics.

Dudley, Cheryl. *Horses that save lives: true stories of physical, emotional and spiritual rescue.* New York: Skyhorse Publishers, 2009.

Contains 24 stories about horses rescuing people, including an Apache teenager who was able to overcome drug addiction from a horse-rescue project; a Vietnam veteran suffering from post-traumatic stress disorder whose work with horses helped emotionally sustain him; and the owner of a miniature horse that serves as a "seeing eye" guide animal.

Eames, Ed and Toni. *Partners in independence: A success story of dogs and the disabled.* Mechanicsburg, PA: Barkleigh Productions, 2004, 2nd ed.

Written by a husband and wife who are both blind, this partly autobiographical work includes chapters on the history of assistance dogs, traveling, caring for these companion animals, and the legal rights of the disabled.

Ensminger, John J. *Service and therapy dogs in American society: science, law and the evolution of canine caregivers*. Springfield, IL: Charles C. Thomas, 2010.

Written by an attorney, this book primarily focuses on the legal rights of service and therapy dog owners in public accommodations and also their protection through other antidiscrimination legislation. The author, who has a therapy dog, also provides some historical background on AAT and service dogs. The work includes extensive bibliographic references and a state-by-state listing of service and therapy dog organizations.

Fine, Aubrey H. and Cynthia J. Eisen. *Afternoons with puppy: inspirations from a therapist and his animals*. West Lafayette, IN: Purdue University Press, 2008.

Although the review words "inspiring" and "heartwarming" have become clichés, this work merits those adjectives. Co-authored by a noted clinical psychologist and a literature professor, this book discusses the ways a variety of animals including dogs, a cockatoo, and even fish can be used in therapeutic settings. The author shows how his animals serve as "co-therapists," providing both quiet comfort and warmth to patients in therapy. The book is dedicated to Puppy, Dr. Fine's late golden retriever, "who more than any other animal opened my eyes to the miracles that can be found in the human/animal bond."

Fine, Aubrey H. *Handbook of animal-assisted therapy: theoretical foundations and guidelines for practice*. Amsterdam; Boston: Elsevier/Academic Press, 2006, 2nd ed.

Edited by the preeminent animal assistance therapist and psychologist, this work contains outstanding background information written by a variety of experts covering the philosophy, practice, and implementation of animal-assisted therapy programs. Special chapters cover children, the elderly, the chronically sick and disabled, and the care and handling of assistance animals. An essential book for any researcher.

Gardner, Nuala. *A friend like Henry: the remarkable true story of an autistic boy and the dog that unlocked his world*. Naperville, IL: Sourcebooks, Inc., 2008.

A touching memoir written by a Scottish woman about how a golden retriever puppy named Henry profoundly affected the life of her son Dale and the rest of their family.

Gross, Patty Dobbs. *The golden bridge: a guide to assistance dogs for children challenged by autism or other developmental disabilities*. West Lafayette, IN: Purdue University Press, 2006.

The author, who founded a nonprofit organization called North Star Foundation that places assistance dogs with children challenged by autism and other disabilities, has written a useful manual for parents and other family members contemplating this type of therapy. The work contains helpful information on many aspects of training and living with assistance dogs and also includes a poignant discussion about the experiences of the author who is the mother of a child with autism.

Joseph, Melissa. *Moments with Baxter: comfort and love from the world's best therapy dog*. San Diego: Sage Press, 2009.

Baxter was a rescue dog who became a certified therapy animal visiting sick individuals in the San Diego Hospice and Palomar Pomerado Hospital. This volume contains 36 stories accompanied by lovely photographs Baxter's profound effect on both the patients and their families.

Katcher, Aaron H. and Alan M. Beck, eds. *New perspectives on our lives with companion animals*. Philadelphia: University of Pennsylvania Press, 1983.

This book contains original and edited papers delivered at the International Conference on the Human-Companion Animal Bond held at the University of Pennsylvania in October 1981. A lengthy section covers the therapeutic uses of companion animals. This work complements Beck and Katcher's more popular later volume, *Between Pets and People* (see above).

Levinson, Boris M. and Gerald P. Mallon. *Pet-oriented child psychotherapy*. Springfield, IL: Charles C Thomas, 2nd edition, rev. and updated, 1997.

This pathbreaking work was written by the psychologist who is credited with starting the field of animal-assisted therapy. Originally published in 1969, this updated and revised edition was edited by a Columbia University professor who has written extensively on the topic. In the preface, he provides very interesting biographical information about Dr. Levinson and the development and growth of animal-assisted therapy.

Long, Lorie. *A dog who's always welcome: assistance and therapy dog trainers teach you how to socialize and train your companion dog*. Hoboken: Wiley, 2008.

Although this book is primarily aimed at dog owners wanting to socialize their pets, the book does contain some interesting chapters on assistance and therapy dogs that may persuade readers to enlist their dogs in such programs.

Lufkin, Elise. *To the rescue: found dogs with a mission*. New York: Skyhorse Publishing, 2009.

A poignant collection of stories about pound and shelter dogs and strays (and also one cat) who are adopted into homes where they are trained to become therapy and service assistance animals. Beautiful photographs by Diane Walker, a nationally known photojournalist, enhance the touching text.

Pavlides, Merope. *Animal-assisted interventions for individuals with autism.* London: Jessica Kingsley, 2008.

Written by a mother of a child with autism, this book discusses a variety of therapeutic approaches including horseback riding, service dogs, and dolphin therapy. She discusses the benefits of these different types of therapy but also notes possible problems with some animal species. Well-written and researched, the book also contains a very useful bibliography.

Pichot, Teri and Marc Coulter. *Animal-assisted brief therapy: a solution-focused approach.* New York: Haworth Press, 2008.

This specialized work aimed at therapists and other mental health professionals recommends specific guidelines in using animal-assisted therapy.

Rivera, Michelle. *On dogs and dying: inspirational stories from hospice hounds.* West Lafayette, IN: Purdue University Press, 2010

In twenty-one stories, an experienced animal therapist chronicles the visits by her two therapy dogs to patients living in a Florida hospice. She also offers tips on training and certifying dogs to be therapy animals.

Sakson, Sharon R. *Paws & effect: the healing power of dogs.* New York: Alyson Books, 2007.

Offering a thumbnail history of dog domestication and the evolution of different breeds, the author of this popular work also provides lovely anecdotes about dogs who have helped war veterans and patients coping with life-threatening illnesses, among other stories. An appendix lists some organizations and a short bibliography includes both print and online sources.

Urichuk, Liana with Dennis Anderson. *Improving mental health through animal-assisted therapy.* Edmonton, Alberta, Canada: The Chimo Project, 2003. This publication can be accessed at http://www.angelfire.com/mh/chimo/pdf/manual_in_single_doc-Nov03.pdf.

The Canadian authors generously posted this manual on the web for non-commercial use. It is primarily geared to mental health professionals and "is based on experiences of people who have incorporated animals into their professions for a variety of purposes."

Wilkes, Jane K. *The role of companion animals in counseling and psychology: discovering their use in the therapeutic process.* Springfield, IL: Charles C. Thomas, 2009.

Another work aimed at mental health professionals, this volume recommends the ways animals can be successfully utilized during therapy sessions and discusses psychological theories pertinent to the human-animal bond.

Wilson, Cindy C. and Dennis C. Turner. *Companion animals in human health.* Thousand Oaks, CA: Sage Publications, 1998.

This informative anthology contains chapters discussing the medical and health benefits derived from pet ownership and companionship. The work also features essays on the history of animal-assisted therapy and discusses specific types of treatment, including equine therapy.

VIDEOS

Ability, not disability
1 videocassette (23 minutes)
Alameda, CA: Latham Foundation, 1975

Filmed at the Cheff Center for the Handicapped, established as the first riding therapy center in the United States in 1970, this short video discusses the therapeutic benefits of riding horses and the Center's instructor-trainee program.

Animal-assisted therapy for young children
1 videorecording (30 minutes)
Macomb, IL: STARnet Regions 1 & II
Center for Best Practices in Early Childhood Education
Western Illinois University, Horrabin Hall 32
1 University Circle, Macomb, IL 61455
(800) 227-7537/(309) 298-1634

This video discusses the positive impact dogs have on children, especially those with disabilities. The video also provides several examples of dogs used in preschool therapeutic settings.

Becoming a R.E.A.D. team
1 videocassette (25 minutes)
Park City, Utah: Main Frame Films (Produced by Intermountain Therapy Animals), 2003
Also check the *Intermountain Therapy Animals* online store for other videos at http://www.therapyanimals.org.

This video discusses the programs of R.E.A.D. (Reading Education Assistance Dogs), an innovative program using dogs to help children in schools and libraries to improve their literacy skills.

Blindness: living fully in a seeing world
1 videodisc (22 minutes)
Sherborn, MA: Aquarius Health Care Videos, 2004

Bill, a blind man with severe allergies, gets help from a service dog with a mind of his own. An equestrian champion continues competitive riding even after going completely blind.

Canine Companions for Independence (four in one) program
1 videocassette (60 minutes)
Santa Rosa: California, Canine Companions for Independence, 1991.
Also check out the Canine Companions for Independence website, which offers several online videos on this web page: http://www.cci.org/site/c.cdKGIRNqEmG/b.4010997/k.C232/Video.htm.

Segments from several television programs featuring dogs who have been trained to do tasks, such as turning off lights, picking up dropped keys, and pulling wheelchairs, to help people with disabilities live more independently.

Dolphin therapy: unique interactions that have life-changing effects on children with disabilities
1 videodisc (26 minutes)
Sherborn, MA: Aquarius Health Care Videos, 2004
Aquarius Health Care Media sells many other videos on animal-assisted therapy at their website, http://www.aquariusproductions.com.

This video examines the effects of dolphin therapy on children with both mental and physical disorders. In one segment, a father brings his autistic son to visit the dolphins to help him develop self-esteem.

Equine assisted therapy: helping build self-esteem and confidence
1 videodisc (30 minutes)
Sherborn, MA: Aquarius Health Care Videos, 2004

This film shows how horses help build self-esteem for riders afflicted with serious emotional problems.

Equine facilitated therapy: a unique therapeutic approach to rehabilitation
1 videorecording (12 minutes)
Woodside, CA: National Center for Equine Facilitated Therapy

This video discusses equine-assisted activity and therapy programs for individuals with neuromuscular and sensory disabilities.

Healing with animals
4 videodiscs
Kelowna, BC; Carson City, NV: Filmwest Associates, 2003
2400 Hayman Road, Kelowna, British Columbia, Canada;
toll-free 1-888-982-FILM (3456)

A 13-part documentary series that explores the many levels at which animals enhance human health: a cat provides "purr-therapy" to a man in pain, and a special canine burn victim brings joy to human burn survivors. This video also shows dogs helping to rehabilitate women in prison and dolphins who swim with autistic kids.

Jenni's journal video essay of a animal therapist
1 videodisc (16 minutes)
Alameda, CA: Latham Foundation, 2005
The Latham Foundation offers many videos on human-animal relationships, in addition to animal-assisted therapy films. http://www.latham.org/videos.asp?Type=Video.

"Jenni Dunn was a therapy dog, living daily for others. From her first days of training, testing, and qualifying as a therapy dog, through the day she was part of a woman's miraculous recovery from coma, Jenni brought joy, hope, and love to countless hospital patients. [Her owner, Linda Dunn] chronicled her adventures in a diary, which has been excerpted in past issues of the Latham Letter."

Just a little hope
1 videocassette (24 minutes)
Alameda, CA: Latham Foundation, 1987

A remarkable story about a man who suffered suicidal depression after surviving kidney failure, two unsuccessful kidney transplants, and three heart attacks. He narrates this personal account of how a psychiatrist-prescribed dog changed his life.

Kerry
1 videocassette (26 minutes)
Walnut Creek, CA: Final Cut Video, 1996
Available from the Latham Foundation, http://www.latham.org/videos.asp?Type=Video.

A documentary about Kerry Knaus-Hardy, a quadriplegic woman who was the first participant in Canine Companions for Independence and a founder of Horseback Outdoor/Recreation and Specialized Equipment and Services (H.O.R.S.E.S., Ltd.), a recreational riding program for individuals with physical disabilities.

Pet-facilitated therapy
1 videocassette (24 minutes)
Alameda, CA: Latham Foundation, 1975.

This video portrays a former patient at Lima State Hospital in Ohio who participated in its unique animal-assisted therapy program. The film recounts his life and attitudes since release.

Pet therapy is making a difference: here's how to do it
1 videocassette
Co-produced by Therapet, Inc., P.O. Box 787, Clark, NJ 07066
phone: 732-602-1112
Discusses an animal-assisted visitation and therapy program in New Jersey.

Prison pet partnerships
1 videocassette (35 minutes)
Alameda, CA: Latham Foundation, 1975

Describes a program at Washington's Purdy Women's Prison in which dogs from humane societies are obedience-trained at the penitentiary and then placed in homes. Both inmates and program administrators describe the benefits of the program.

Prison Pups
1 videocassette (58 minutes)
Watertown, MA: Documentary Educational Resources, 2006

Starting in the late 1990s, an animal-assistance therapy group called NEADS (National Education for Assistance Dog Service) began working with prisoners in Massachusetts to help train dogs to assist people with disabilities. The NEADS director was initially skeptical, but she later proudly declared that the best-trained and most loving dogs came from this program. While the film poignantly shows the remarkable relationship that can develop between the dogs and their prison trainers, it does not gloss over problems, for example, inmates removed from the project for disciplinary infractions and the resentment of nonparticipating prisoners. Nevertheless, the film mostly discusses the profound ways this program helped change the lives of some inmates, their families, and, especially, the disabled people who eventually adopted the dogs.

Service, therapy and emotional support: animal legal protections for individuals with disabilities
2 sound recordings (160 minutes).
New York: City Bar Center for CLE, 2003

A panel discussion held on June 3, 2003, to discuss the legal issues surrounding service animals, emotional support animals, and therapy animals. Includes definitions, the impact of the Americans with Disabilities Act, and what constitutes discrimination.

Teamwork: a dog training video for people with disabilities
1 videodisc (105 minutes)
Tucson, AZ: TopDog Productions, 2003.

This instructional video shows people with disabilities the methods for training their dogs. These techniques are applicable for people who use canes, crutches, and walkers, and for individuals in wheelchairs.

Through a dog's eyes
1 videodisc (60 minutes)
Melbourne, FL: PBS Home Video, 2010
(PO Box 609 Melbourne, FL 32902-0609; toll-free 1-800-531-4727)

Shown in prime time on PBS during the spring of 2010, this documentary narrates poignant stories of people with disabilities and the way they develop close relationships with service dogs. (See companion volume in "Boths" section.)

Tuskegee behavior test for selecting therapy dogs
1 videocassette (23 minutes), 1993.
Tuskegee, AL: Tuskegee University School of Veterinary Medicine, Media Center, 1993.

Describes the canine behavior test developed at Tuskegee University School of Veterinary Medicine, focusing on how dogs interact with owners and strangers. The video is used for screening dogs for visits to hospital patients and also nursing home residents.

Journal and Other Articles

Please note: The following two journals specialize in coverage of the human-animal bond and have published numerous articles on animal-assisted therapy. The following bibliography lists only some of these article titles.

Anthrozoos (ISSN: 0892-7936; Online ISSN: 1753-0377) is the official quarterly journal of the International Society for Anthrozoology. Founded in 1987, this peer-reviewed journal addresses "the characteristics and consequences of interactions and relationships between people and non-human animals across areas as varied as anthropology, ethology, medicine, psychology, veterinary medicine and zoology."

Society & Animals (ISSN:1063-1119; E-ISSN:1568-5306), a quarterly, publishes "studies that describe and analyze our experiences of non-human animals from the perspective of various disciplines within both the social sciences (e.g., psychology, sociology, anthropology, political science) and

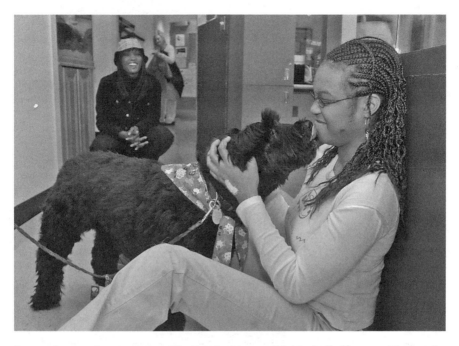

Jane, a therapy dog, expresses affection to 14 year-old Alexia Godfrey, a patient at the Albany (New York) Medical Center, as her mother looks on. (AP Photo/Tim Roske)

humanities (e.g., history, literary criticism). The journal specifically deals with subjects such as human-animal interactions in various settings (animal cruelty and the therapeutic uses of animals), among many other topics.

Children and Adolescents

Abraham, Shalev & Ben-Mordehai, Dror. (1996). Snakes: Interactions with children with disabilities and the elderly—some psychological considerations. *Anthrozoos*, 9(4), 182–187.

Bardill, N. & Hutchinson, S. (1997). Animal-assisted therapy with hospitalized adolescents. *Journal of Child & Adolescent Psychiatric Nursing*, 10(1), 17–24.

Bodmer, N. M. (1998). Impact of pet ownership on the well-being of adolescents with few familial resources. In Cindy Wilson and Dennis Turner (eds.) *Companion Animals in Human Health*. Thousand Oaks, CA: Sage, pp. 237–247.

Flom, Barbara L. (2005). Counseling with pocket pets: using small animals in elementary counseling programs. *Professional School Counseling*, 8(5), 469–471.

Heimlich, Kathryn. (2001). Animal-assisted therapy and the severely disabled child: a quantitative study. *Journal of Rehabilitation* 67(4), 48–54.

Kirton, Adam, et al. (2004). Seizure-alerting and response behaviors in dogs living with epileptic children. *Neurology* 62, 2303–2305.

Kruger, Katherine, Trachtenberg, S. &Serpell, J. A. (2004). Can animals help humans heal? Animal-assisted interventions in adolescent mental health. http://research.vet.upenn.edu/Portals/36/media/CIAS_AAI_white_paper.pdf.

Mallon, Gerald P. (1994). Cow as co-therapist: Utilization of farm animals as therapeutic aids with children in residential treatment. *Child and Adolescent Social Work Journal* 11(6), 455–474.

Mallon, Gerald P. (1994). Some of the best therapists are dogs. *Child and Youth Care Forum* 23(2), 89–101.

Mallon, Gerald P. (1992). Utilization of animals as therapeutic adjuncts with children and youth: A review of the literature. *Child and Youth Care Forum* 21(1), 53–67.

Nathanson, D. E. (1998). Long-term effectiveness of dolphin-assisted therapy for children with severe disabilities. *Anthrozoos* 11, 22–32.

Nebbe, L. L. (1991). The human-animal bond and the elementary school counselor. *School Counselor* 38(5), 362–371.

Poresky, Robert & Hendrix, C. (1990). Differential effects of pet presence and pet bonding in young children. *Psychological Reports* 67(1), 51–54.

Reichert, E. (1998). Individual counseling for sexually abused children : A role for animals and storytelling. *Child and Adolescent Social Work Journal* 15(3), 177–185.

Ricard, Marcelle & Allard, L. (1993). The reaction of 9- to 10 month-old infants to an unfamiliar animal. *Journal of Genetic Psychology*, 154, 5–16.

Riegger, M. H. & Guntzelman, J. (1990). Prevention and amelioration of stress and consequences of interaction between children and dogs. *Journal of the American Veterinary Medical Association* 196(11) 1781–1785.

Robin, Michael & ten Bensel, Robert (1985). Pets and the socialization of children. *Marriage and Family Review* 8(3/4), 63–78.

Rost, Detlef H. & Hartmann, Anette (1994). Children and their pets. *Anthrozoos* 7(4), 242–254.

Sams, M. J., Fortney, E. V. and Willenbring, S. (2006). Occupational therapy incorporating animals for children with autism: A pilot investigation. *American Journal of Occupational Therapy* 60(3), 268–274.

Triebenbacher, Sandra L. (1998). Pets as transitional objects: Their role in children's emotional development. *Psychological Reports* 82(1), 191–200.

Vidovic, V. V., Stectic, V. V. & Bratko, D. (1999). Pet ownership, type of pet and socioemotional development of school children. *Anthrozoos* 12(4), 211–217.

The Elderly

Banks, Marian R. & Banks, William A. (2005). The effects of group and individual animal-assisted therapy on loneliness in residents of long-term care facilities. *Anthrozoos*, 18(4), 396–408.

Batson, Kathryn, McCabe, Barbara W., Baun, Mara M. & Wilson, Carol (1998) The effect of a therapy dog on socialization and physiological indicators of stress in persons diagnosed with Alzheimer's disease. In Cindy Wilson & Dennis Turner, (eds.), *Companion Animals in Human Health.* Thousand Oaks, CA: Sage Publications. 203–215.

Baun, Mara M. (2003). Companion animals and persons with dementia of the Alzheimer's type. *American Behavioral Scientist* 47(1), 42–51.

Bernstein, P. I. , Friedmann, Ericka,& Malaspina, A. (2000). Animal-assisted therapy enhances resident social interaction and initiation in long-term care facilities. *Anthrozoos* 13(4), 213–224.

Beyersdorfer, P. & Birkenhauer, D. M. (1990). The therapeutic use of pets on an Alzheimer's unit. *American Journal of Alzheimer's Care and Related Disorders and Research* 5, 13–17.

Boldt, Margaret A. & Dellmann-Jenkins, Mary (1992). The impact of companion animals in later life and considerations for practice. *Journal of Applied Gerontology* 11, 228–239.

Brickel, C. M. (1979). The therapeutic roles of cat mascots with a hospital-based geriatric population. *The Gerontologist* 19(4) 368–372.

Calvert, Melissa M. (1989). Human-pet interaction and loneliness: A test of concepts from Roy's adaptation model. *Nursing Science Quarterly* 2(4), 194–202.

Churchill, M. Safaoui, J., McCabe, B. & Baun, M. M. (1999). Using a therapy dog to alleviate the agitation and desocialization behavior of people with Alzheimer's disease. *Journal of Psychosocial Nursing and Mental Health Services*, 37(4), 16–22.

Colby, Patricia M. & Sherman, Angela (2002). Attachment styles impact on pet visitation effectiveness. *Anthrozoos* 15(2), 150–165.

Crowley-Robinson, P. & Blackshaw, J. K. (1998). Pet ownership and health status of the elderly in the community. *Anthrozoos* 11(3), 168–171.

Crowley-Robinson, P., Fenwick, D. C. & Blackshaw, J.K (1996). A long-term study of elderly people in nursing homes with visiting and resident dogs. *Applied Animal Behaviour Science* 47, 137–148.

Dernbicki, D. & Anderson, J. (1996). Pet ownership may be a factor in the improved health of the elderly. *Journal of Nutrition for the Elderly* 15, 15–31.

DeSchriver, M. & Riddick, Carol (1990). Effects of watching aquariums on elders' stress. *Anthrozoos* 4(1), 44–48.

Fick, K. M. (1993). The influence of an animal on social interactions of nursing home residents in a group setting. *American Journal of Occupational Therapy* 47(6), 529–534.

Francis, Gloria, Turner, J. T. & Johnson, S. B. (1985). Domestic animal visitation as therapy with adult home residents. *International Journal of Nursing Studies* 22, 201–206.

Fritz, C. L., Farver, T. B., Hart, L. A. & Kass, P. H. (1996). Companion animals and the psychological health of Alzheimer's patients' caregivers. *Psychological Reports* 78, 467–481.

Fritz, C. L., Farver, T. B., Kass, P. H. & Hart, L. A. (1995). Association with companion animals and the expression of noncognitive symptoms in Alzheimer's patients. *Journal of Nervous and Mental Disease* 183(7), 459–463.

Gammonley, Judith & Yates, Judy (1991). Pet projects: animal assisted therapy in nursing homes. *Journal of Gerontological Nursing* 17(12), 12–15.

Garrity, Thomas F. et al. (1989). Pet ownership and attachment as supportive factors in the health of the elderly. *Anthrozoos*, 3(1), 35–44.

Greer, Kari L., Pustay, Karen A. Zaun, Tracy C., & Coppens, Patrick (2001). A comparison of the effects of toys versus live animals on the communication of patients with dementia of the Alzheimer's type. *Clinical Gerontologist* 24 (3/4), 157–182.

Hendy, Helen M. (1987). Effects of pet and/ or people visits on nursing home residents. *International Journal of Aging and Human Development* 25, 279–291.

Jessen, J., Cardiello, F. & Baun, M. M. (1996). Avian companionship in alleviation of depression, loneliness, and low morale of older adults in skilled rehabilitation units. *Psychological Reports* 78, 339–348.

Johnson, R. A., Odendaal, J. S. & Meadows, R. L. (2002). Animal assisted intervention research: Issues and answers. *Western Journal of Nursing Research* 24(4), 422–440.

Kongable, L. G. and Buckwalter, K. C. (1990). Pet therapy for Alzheimer's patients: A survey. *Journal of Long-Term Care Administration* 18(3), 17–21.

Kramer, Stephen C. (2009). Comparison of the effect of human interaction, animal-assisted therapy, and AIBO-assisted therapy on long-term care residents with dementia. *Anthrozoos*, 22(1), 43–58.

Levinson, Boris (1970). Nursing home pets: A psychological adventure for the clients. Parts 1 and 2. *National Humane Review* 58, 6–8, 14–16, and 59.

Levinson, Boris (1969). Pets and old age. *National Humane Review* 53, 364–368.

Lutwack-Bloom, Patricia, Wijewickrama, Rohan & Betsy Smith (2005). Effects of pets versus people visits with nursing home residents. *Journal of Gerontological Social Work*, 44(3–4), 123–160.

Manor, Wendy (1991). Alzheimer's patients and their caregivers: the role of the human-animal bond. *Holistic Nursing Practice* 5(2), 32–37.

McCabe, B. W., Baun, M. M, Speich, D., & Agarwal, S. (2002). A resident dog in the Alzheimer's special care unit. *Western Journal of Nursing Research*, 24 (6), 684–696.

Odendaal, J. S. (2000). Animal assisted therapy—magic or medicine? *Journal of Psychosomatic Research*, 49, 275–280.

Ory, M. G. & Goldberg, E. L. (1983). Pet possession and well-being in elderly women. *Research on Aging*, 5(3), 389–409.

Perelle, Ira B. & Granville, Diane A. (1993). Assessment of the effectiveness of a pet-facilitated therapy program in a nursing home setting. *Society and Animals* 1, 91–100.

Raina, P., Waltner-Toews, B. et al. (1999). Influence of companion animals on the physical and psychological health of older people: an analysis of a one-year longitudinal study. *Journal of the American Geriatrics Society*, 47(3), 323–329.

Savishinsky, J. (1985). Pets and family relationships among nursing home residents. *Marriage and Family Review*, 8(3–4), 109–134.

Siegel, Judith M. (1990). Stressful life events and use of physician services among the elderly: The moderating role of pet ownership. *Journal of Personality and Social Psychology*, 58(6), 1081–1086.

Winkler, A., Fairnie, H., Gericevich, F., & Long, M. (1989). The impact of a resident dog on an institution for the elderly: Effects of perceptions on social interaction. *The Gerontologist*, 29(2), 216–223.

Psychotherapy

Allen, L. & Burdon, R. (1982). The clinical significance of pets in a psychiatric community residence. *American Journal of Social Psychiatry* 6, 722–728.

Altschuler, E. L. (1999). Pet-facilitated therapy for posttraumatic stress disorder. *Annals of Clinical Psychiatry* 11, 29–230.

Barker, S. B. & Dawson, K. S. (1998). Effects of animal-assisted therapy on anxiety ratings of hospitalized psychiatric patients. *Psychiatric Services* 49, 797–801.

Beck, Alan M., Seraydarian, L. & Hunter, G. F. (1986). The use of animals in the rehabilitation of psychiatric inpatients. *Psychological Reports* 8, 63–66.

Corson, Samuel A. & Corson, Elizabeth O. (1980). Pet animals as nonverbal communication mediators in psychotherapy in institutional settings. In Samuel A Corson & Elizabeth O. Corson, eds., *Ethology and Nonverbal Communication in Mental Health*. Oxford: Pergamon Press, 83–110.

Corson, Samuel A, Corson, Elizabeth O., Gwynne, P. H. & Arnold, L. B. (1977). Pet dogs as nonverbal communication links in hospital psychiatry. *Comprehensive Psychiatry* 18(1), 61–72.

Corson, S., & Corson, E. (1978). Pets as mediators of therapy. *Current Psychiatric Theories* 18, 195–205.

Fine, Aubrey H. (2006). Incorporating animal-assisted therapy into psychotherapy: guidelines and suggestions for therapists. In Aubrey H. Fine, ed., *Handbook on Animal-Assisted Therapy: Theoretical Foundations and Guidelines for Practice*. San Diego: Academic Press. (2nd ed.), pp. 167–206.

Friedmann, E. & Thomas, S. A. (1995). Pet ownership, social support and one-year survival after acute myocardial infarction in the Cardiac Arrhythmia Suppression Trial (CAST). *American Journal of Cardiology* 76, 1213–1217.

Haughie, E., Milne, D. & Elliott, V. (1992). An evaluation of companion pets with elderly psychiatric patients. *Behavioural Psychotherapy* 20, 367–372.

Kruger, K. A. & Serpell, J. A. (2006). Animal-assisted interventions in mental health. In Aubrey H. Fine (ed.), *Handbook on Animal-Assisted Therapy* (2nd ed.), San Diego: Academic Press, pp. 21–38.

Levinson, Boris (1962). The dog as co-therapist. *Mental Hygiene* 46, 59–65.

Levinson, Boris (1964). Pets: A special technique in child psychotherapy. *Mental Hygiene* 48, 243–248.

Levinson, Boris (1965). Pet psychotherapy: Use of household pets in the treatment of behavior disorder in childhood. *Psychological Reports* 17, 695–698.

Levinson, Boris (1968). Interpersonal relationships between pets and human beings. In Michael.W. Fox, (ed.), *Abnormal Behavior In Animals*. Philadelphia: W. B. Saunders. pp. 504–522.

Levinson, Boris (1969). Household pets in residential schools. *Mental Hygiene* 52, 411–414.

Levinson, Boris (1971). Household pets in training schools serving delinquent children *Psychological Reports* 28, 475–481.

Marr, C. A. et al. (2000). Animal-assisted therapy in psychiatric rehabilitation. *Anthrozoos* 13(1), 43–47.

Motomura, N., Yagi, T., & Ohyama, H. (2004). Animal-assisted therapy for people with dementia. *Psychogeriatrics* 4, 40–42.

Parshall, D. P. (2003). Research and reflection: animal-assisted therapy in mental health settings. *Counseling and Values* 48, 47–56.

Sacks, Anita. (2008). The therapeutic use of pets in private practice. *British Journal of Psychotherapy* 24(4), 501–521.

Siegal, A. (1962). Reaching the severely withdrawn through pet therapy. *American Journal of Psychiatry* 118, 1045–1048.

Villalta-Gil, V. et al. (2009). Dog-assisted therapy in the treatment of chronic schizophrenia inpatients. *Anthrozoos* 22 (2), 149–159.

Wells, E. S., Rosen, L. W. & Walshaw, S. (1997). Use of feral cats in psychotherapy. *Anthrozoos* 10, 125–130.

Wisdom, J. P., Saedi, G. A. & Green, C. A. (2009). Another breed of "service" animals: STARS study findings about pet ownership and recovery from serious mental illness. *American Journal of Orthopsychiatry* 79(3), 430–436.

Service Animals

Allen, Karen & Blascovich, James (1996). The value of service dogs for people with severe ambulatory difficulties. *Journal of the American Medical Association* 275, 1001–1006.

Camp, Mary M. (2001). The use of service dogs as an adaptive strategy: A qualitative study. *American Journal of Occupational Therapy* 55(5), 509–517.

Coppinger, Raymond, Coppinger, L. & Skillings, E. (1998). Observations on assistance dog training and use. *Journal of Applied Animal Welfare Science* 1, 133–144.

Deshen, S. & Deshen, H. (1989). On social aspects of the usage of guide-dogs and long-canes. *Sociological Review* 37(1), 89–103.

Duncan, Susan L. (1998). The importance of training standards and policy for service animals. In Cindy Wilson and Dennis Turner, eds., *Companion Animals in Human Health*. Thousand Oaks CA: Sage Publications, pp. 251–266.

Eames, Ed & Eames, Toni (1996). Economic consequences of partnerships with service dogs. *Disability Studies Quarterly* 16(4), 19–25.

Eames, Ed, Eames, Toni & Diament, Sara (2001). Guide dog teams in the United States: annual number trained and active, 1993–1999. *Journal of Visual Impairment & Blindness* 95(7), 434–437.

Eddy, Jane, Hart, Lynette A. & Boltz, R. P. (1988). The effects of service dogs on social acknowledgments of people in wheelchairs. *Journal of Psychology* 122, 39–45.

Fairman, Stacey K. & Huebner, Ruth A. (2000). Service dogs: A compensatory resource to improve function. *Occupational Therapy in Health Care* 13(2), 41–52.

Frei, C. E. (1998). Providing "Paws" for independence. *Exceptional Parent*, 68–73.

Gaunet, F. (2008). How do guide dogs of blind owners and pet dogs of sighted owners (Canis familiaris) ask their owners for food? *Animal Cognition*, 11(3), 475–483.

Hart, Lynette A., Hart, Benjamin & Bergin, Bonita (1987). Socializing effects of service dogs for people with disabilities. *Anthrozoos* 1(1), 41–44.

Hart, Lynette A, Zasloff, R. L. & Benfatto, A M. (1995). The pleasures and problems of hearing dog ownership. *Psychological Reports* 77 (3), 969–970.

Hart, Lynette A, Zasloff, R & Benfatto, A. M. (1996). The socializing role of hearing dogs. *Applied Animal Behaviour Science* 47, 7–15.

Lane, D. R., McNicholas, J. & Collis, Glyn M. (1998). Dogs for the disabled: Benefits to recipients and welfare of the dog. *Applied Animal Behavioural Science* 59, 49–60.

Mader, Bonnie, Hart, Lynette A & Bergin, Bonita (1989). Social acknowledgements for children with disabilities: Effects of service dogs. *Child Development* 60, 1528–1534.

Miura, Ayaka, Tanida, Hajime & Bradshaw, John W.S (1998). Provision of service dogs for people with mobility disabilities. *Anthrozoos* 11(2), 105–108.

Miura, Ayaka, Bradshaw, John W. S. & Tanida, Hajime (2002). Attitudes toward assistance dogs in Japan and the UK: a comparison of college students studying animal care. *Anthrozoos* 15(3), 227–242.

Modlin, Susan (2000). Service dogs as interventions: State of the science. *Rehabilitation Nursing* 25(6), 212–219.

Modlin, Susan (2001). From puppy to service dog: Raising service dogs for the rehabilitation team. *Rehabilitation Nursing* 26(1), 12–17.

Murphy, J. A. (1998). Describing categories of temperament in potential guide dogs for the blind. *Applied Animal Behaviour Science* 58(1–2), 163–178.

Nicholson, J., Kemp-Wheeler, S. & Griffiths, D. (1995). Distress arising from the end of a guide dog partnership. *Anthrozoos*, 8(2), 100–110.

Steffens, Melanie C. & Bergler, R. (1998). Blind people and their dogs: An empirical study on changes in everyday life, in self-experience, and in communication. In C. C. Wilson and D. C.Turner (eds.) *Companion animals in human health*. Thousand Oaks, CA: Sage Publications. pp. 149–157.

Weiss, E. (2002). Selecting shelter dogs for service dog training. *Journal of Applied Animal Welfare Science* 5, 43–62.

Wiggett-Barnard, C. & Steel, H. (2008). The experience of owning a guide dog. *Disability and Rehabilitation: An International Multidisciplinary Journal*, 30(14), 1014–1026.

Therapeutic Horseback Riding/Dolphin Therapy

All, Anita, Loving, Gary & Crane, Laura L. (1999). Animals, horseback riding, and implications for rehabilitation therapy. *Journal of Rehabilitation* 65(3), 49–57.

Benda, W., McGibbon, N. H. & Grant, K. L. (2003). Improvements in muscle symmetry in children with cerebral palsy after equine-assisted therapy. *Journal of Alternative and Complementary Medicine* 9, 817–825.

Bertoti, D. B. (1988). Effects of therapeutic horseback riding on posture in children with cerebral palsy. *Physical Therapy* 68, 1505–1512.

Biery, Martha J. (1985). Riding and the handicapped. *Veterinary Clinics of North America Small Animal Practice* 15(2), 345–354.

Biery, Martha J. & Kauffman, Nancy (1989). The effects of therapeutic horseback riding on balance. *Adapted Physical Activity Quarterly* 6, 220–229.

Bizub, A. L., Joy, A. & Davidson, L. (2003). It's like being in another world: Demonstrating the benefits of therapeutic horseback riding for individuals with psychiatric disability. *Psychiatric Rehabilitation Journal* 26, 377–384.

Brensing, Karsten (2005). Expert-Statement Subject: "Swim with the dolphin programs" and "Dolphin-assisted therapy." Accessed at http://www.sccptiques.qc.ca/dictionnaire/userfiles/file/dat.pdf.

Casady, R. L. & Nichols-Larsen, D. S. (2004). The effect of hippotherapy on ten children with cerebral palsy. *Pediatric Physical Therapy* 16, 165–172.

Cawley, Roger, Cawley, Doreen & Retter, Kristen (1994). Therapeutic horseback riding and self-concept in adolescents with special educational needs. *Anthrozoos* 7(2), 129–134.

Cumella, Edward J. (2003). Question: Is equine therapy useful in the treatment of eating disorders? *Eating Disorders* 11(2), 143–147.

Fitzpatrick, J. C. & Tebay, Jean M. (1997). Hippotherapy and therapeutic riding. In Cindy C. Wilson & Dennis C. Turner, eds., *Companion Animals in Human Health*. Thousand Oaks, CA: Sage Publications, pp. 41–58.

Funk, Marcia S. M. & Smith, Betsy A. (2000). Occupational therapists and therapeutic riding. *Anthrozoos* 13(3), 174–181.

Hart, Lynette A. (1992). Therapeutic riding: Assessing human versus horse effects. *Anthrozoos* 5(3), 138–139.

Land, Gary, Errington-Povalac, Emily & Paul, Stanley (2001). The effects of therapeutic riding on sitting posture in individuals with disabilities. *Occupational Therapy in Health Care* 14(1), 1–12.

Marino, L. (1998). "Dolphin-assisted therapy: flawed data, flawed conclusions." *Anthrozoos* 11(4), 194–200

McCowan, Lida (1984). "Equestrian therapy." In Phil Arkow, ed., *Dynamic Relationships in Practice: Animals In the Helping Professions*. Alameda, CA: Latham Foundation.

Meinersmann, K. M. (2008). Equine-facilitated psychotherapy with adult female survivors of abuse. *Journal of Psychosocial Nursing and Mental Health Services* 46(12), 37–42.

Nathanson, D. E. (1998). Long-term effectiveness of dolphin-assisted therapy for children with severe disabilities. *Anthrozoos* 11(1), 22–32.

Pavlides, M. (2008). "Dolphin Therapy" In Pavlides, M., ed. *Animal-assisted interventions for individuals with autism*. London: Jessica Kingsley Publishers, pp. 160–185.

Rothe, E. Q. et al. (2005). From kids and horses: Equine-facilitated psychotherapy for children. *International Journal of Clinical and Health Psychology* 5 (3), 373–383.

Smith, Betsy (2003). "The discovery and development of dolphin-assisted therapy". In T. Frohoff and B. Peterson (eds.), *Between species: celebrating the dolphin-human bond*. San Francisco: Sierra Club Books. pp. 239–246.

Vidrine, Maureen, Owen-Smith, Patti & Faulkner,Priscilla (2002). Equine-facilitated group psychotherapy: Applications for therapeutic vaulting. *Issues in Mental Health Nursing* 23(6), 587–603.

General and Miscellaneous Articles on Animal-Assisted Therapy

Adamle, Kathleen M. (2009). Evaluating college student interest in pet therapy. *Journal of American College Health* 57(5), 545–549.

Adams, D. L. (1997). Animal-assisted enhancement of speech therapy: A case study. *Anthrozoos* 10(1), 53–56.

Adams, Kristina (2004). *Brief information resource on assistance animals for the disabled*. Primarily citations from the Agricola database; also lists web resources and a glossary of the various categories for assistance and service animals. Accessed at http://www.nal..usda.gov/awic/companimals/assist.htm.

Anthrozoology: Research in human-animal interaction (2008). Contains annotated citations to academic journals on a variety of topics, including animal-assisted therapy. Accessed at http://www.anthrozoology.org/pdf/anthrozoology.pdf.

Baranauckas, Carla (2009). Exploring the health benefits of pets. *New York Times* Section D5 (October 6).

Barker, Sandra B. et al. (2003). Benefits of interacting with companion animals: a bibliography of articles published in refereed journals during the past 5 years. *American Behavioral Scientist* 47(1), 94–99.

Beck, Alan M. & Aaron Katcher (2003). Future directions in human-animal bond. *American Behavioral Scientist* 47(1), 79–93.

Behm, Leslie M. (2004). Human-animal bond, animal therapy, and service animals. [Annotated bibliography on these topics] Chicago, IL: Medical Library Association, MLA Bibkit#10. Access publication list at http://www.mlanet.org.

Brodie, S. J., F. C. Biley, et al. (2002). An exploration of the potential risks associated with using pet therapy in healthcare settings. *Journal of Clinical Nursing* 11(4), 444–456.

Brody, Jane E. (1998). Staying healthy with fins, fur and feathers. *New York Times* Section F7, (June 23).

Burke, Sarah (1992). In the presence of animals. *U.S. News and World Report* 112 (February 24), 64–65.

Canine candy stripers (2001). *Time* 158, (August 6), 52–53.

Curtis, P. (1981). Animals are good for the handicapped, perhaps all of us. *Smithsonian* 12(4), 49–57.

Eachus, P. (2001). Pets, people and robots: the role of companion animals and robopets in the promotion of health and well-being. *International Journal of Health Promotion & Education* 39(1), 7–13. [ISSN 1463–5240]

Fields-Meyer, Thomas & Mandel, Susan (2006). Healing hounds. *People* July 17, 101–102.

Fischman, Josh (2005). Pet Prescription. *U.S. News and World Report* 139 (22), 72–74, December 12.

Ford, B. (1976). Pet therapy: my dog the analyst. *Science Digest* 79, 58–64.

Hatch, Alison (2007). The view from all fours: a look at an animal-assisted activity program from the animals' perspective. *Anthrozoos* 20 (1), 37–50.

Hines, Linda M. (2003). Historical perspectives on the human-animal bond. *American Behavioral Scientist* 47(1), 7–15.

Huebscher, R. (2000). Pets and animal-assisted therapy. *Nurse Practitioner Forum* 11(1), 1–4.

Lorber, Jane (2010). For the battle-scarred, comfort at leash's end: Service dogs used in post-trauma cases. *New York Times* Section A19, (April 4).

Monkeys assisting people with disabilities: a bibliography (2008). [Useful specialized bibliography compiled at the National Primate Research Center, University of Wisconsin-Milwaukee] Accessed at http://pin.primate.wisc.edu/infoserv/askprim/helpcit.html.

Serpell, J. (1991). Beneficial effects of pet ownership on some aspects of human health and behavior. *Journal of the Royal Society of Medicine* 84(12), 717–720.

Shallcross, Lynne (2008). Four legs doing good. *Washingtonian* 44(3), December, 185.

Whittington, Anne E. (2008). 'Is Karl in?': Paws that heal. *American Journal of Nursing* 108(7), 31–34.

ORGANIZATIONS

Please note: Website contents and URLs frequently change. If you can't find the organization under the current address, please do a Google search on the organizational name.

American Hippotherapy Association

9919 Towne Road
Carmel, Indiana 46032
Phone: 877-851-4592
http://www.americanhippotherapyassociation.org

This organization "promotes the use of the movement of the horse as a treatment strategy in physical, occupational and speech-language therapy sessions for people living with disabilities. Hippotherapy has been shown to improve muscle tone, balance, posture, coordination, motor development as well as emotional well-being." The membership includes physical, occupational, and speech-language therapists and others interested in the benefits offered in equine therapy.

American Humane Association (AHA)

Animal-Assisted Therapy Program
63 Inverness Drive East
Englewood, CO 80112
Phone: 800-227-4645
http://www.americanhumane.org

Headquartered in the Denver, Colorado area, this program collaborates with individuals and organizations to help them conduct effective animal-assisted therapy. AHA has more than 200 handler-animal teams serving 50 facilities in the Denver area. Besides serving hospitals, nursing homes, rehabilitation centers, group homes, mental health centers and schools, this program also works with a homeless shelter, an HIV clinic and a juvenile correctional facility.

Assistance Dogs of America, Inc.

8806 State Rte. 64
Swanton, OH 43558
Phone: 419-825-3622
http://www.adai.org

This Ohio-based organization trains service and therapy dogs to assist children and adults with disabilities and has helped more than 150 individuals in the last few decades. The canine companions visit school children and nursing home residents suffering from a variety of disabilities, including muscular dystrophy, spina bifida, cerebral palsy, and spinal cord injuries.

Assistance Dogs International

P.O. Box 5174
Santa Rosa, California 95402
Phone: 707-545-3647
http://www.assistancedogsinternational.org

A coalition of not-for-profit organizations that train and place assistance dogs. Aims to improve the areas of training, placement, and utilization of assistance dogs. Member organizations meet regularly to share ideas about educating the public about assistance dogs, the legal rights of people with disabilities partnered with these canines, and setting standards and ethical guidelines for the training of these dogs.

Bright and Beautiful Therapy Dogs

80 Powder Mill Road
Morris Plains, NJ 07950
Phone: 973-292-3316 ; Toll-free 888-PET-5770
http://www.golden-dogs.org

"Evaluates, tests, trains, qualifies and supports therapy dogs for the purpose of giving loving and empathic support in nursing homes, hospitals, psychiatric wards and other facilities where emotional service dogs are indispensable. These dogs, once they qualify to become members of The Bright and Beautiful Therapy Dogs, Inc., will receive many benefits including primary accident and liability insurance within the U.S., therapy dog equipment, post card mailings and quarterly newsletters."

Canine Companions for Independence

P.O. Box 446
Santa Rosa, CA 95402-0446
Phone: 800-572-2275
http://www.caninecompanions.org

Provides trained dogs to individuals with disabilities and offers four types of canine companions:

- Hearing dogs trained to alert the hearing-impaired to sounds such as doorbells, smoke alarms, a child crying or timers on microwave ovens.
- Companion dogs used for children and adults with disabilities and people with developmental disabilities.
- Service dogs trained to provide physical assistance, such as retrieving dropped objects, operating elevator buttons and light switches, etc.
- Facility dogs placed with professionals in facilities where interaction with a dog will be beneficial to the mental or physical health of those in their care.

Canine Therapy Corps

1700 West Irving Park Road, Suite 311
Chicago, Illinois 60613
Phone: 773-404-6467
http://www.caninetherapycorps.org

A Chicago-based network of volunteers and their certified therapy dogs, this organization offers rehabilitative therapy for people with physical and psychological problems.

Delta Society

875 124th Ave. NE, Ste. 101
Bellevue, WA 98005
Phone: 425-679-5500
http://www.deltasociety.org

"The mission of Delta Society is to help lead the world in advancing human health and well-being through positive interactions with animals. We help people throughout the world become healthier and happier by incorporating therapy, service and companion animals into their lives." Trains and registers volunteers to provide animal-assisted activities and/or therapy in their Pet Partners program. The organization operates a National Service Dog Center serving people with disabilities via a website.

Helping Hands

541 Cambridge Street
Boston, MA 02134
Phone: 617-787-4419
http://www.monkeyhelpers.org

This national nonprofit organization serves quadriplegic and other people with severe spinal cord injuries or mobility impairments by providing highly trained monkeys to assist with daily activities. The organization raises and trains monkeys to act as live-in companions who—over a 20- to 30-year period—help provide independence and companionship to individuals with disabilities.

Also educates thousands of young people annually through the Spinal Cord Injury Prevention Program (SCIPP), which teaches "preventive measures for safety awareness" and "heightens sensitivity to the challenges of being disabled, and promotes understanding of the human-animal bond."

International Association of Human-Animal Interaction Organizations

c/o SCAS-UK
10B Leny Road
Callander
FK17 8BA
Scotland, United Kingdom
http://www.iahaio.org

Founded in 1990, this umbrella international organization gathers together national associations and related organizations interested in advancing the understanding and appreciation of the link between animals and humans.

The Association's main role is to provide a coordinating structure between all member countries. In addition, this international organization has established a series of awards to acknowledge contributions made by individuals or institutions in the study of the human-companion animal relationship. These awards include the IAHAIO "Pets in Cities" and "Distinguished Scholar" Awards, which are presented every three years.

International Association of Assistance Dog Partners

c/o Carol Schilling
P.O. Box 235
Troy, MI 48099-0235
Phone: 888-544-2237 (USA / North America)
http://www.iaadp.org

A non-profit organization launched in 1993 at the joint Delta Society and Assistance Dogs International conference "to establish an independent cross disability consumer organization that could represent all Assistance Dog Partners (not just one faction) and advance consumer interests in the assistance dog field."

The mission: to provide assistance dog partners with a voice in the assistance dog field; to enable those partnered with guide dogs, hearing dogs and service dogs to work together on issues of mutual concern; to foster the disabled person/ assistance dog partnership for people with disabilities working with guide, hearing and service dogs.

Intermountain Therapy Animals

P.O. Box 17201
Salt Lake City, Utah 84117
Phone: 801-272-3439
http://www.therapyanimals.org/READ

"The mission of the R.E.A.D.® program is to improve the literacy skills of children through the assistance of registered therapy teams as literacy mentors. The Reading Education Assistance Dogs (R.E.A.D.) program improves children's reading and communication skills by employing a powerful method: reading to a dog . . . but not just any dog. R.E.A.D. dogs are registered therapy animals who volunteer with their owner/handlers as a team, going to schools, libraries and many other settings as reading companions for children."

R.E.A.D. was launched in 1999 as the first comprehensive literacy program built around the unique idea of children reading to dogs.

Latham Foundation

Latham Plaza Building
1826 Clement Avenue
Alameda, CA 94501
Phone: 1-510-521-0920
http://www.Latham.org

Founded in 1918, this Foundation serves as a clearinghouse for information about humane issues and activities; the Human Companion Animal Bond (HCAB); animal-assisted therapy; and the connections between child and animal abuse and other forms of violence. The Foundation is a producer and distributor of videos, including many documentaries on animal-therapy programs.

National Center for Equine-Facilitated Therapy (NCEFT)

880 Runnymede Road
Woodside CA 94062
Phone: 650-851-2271
Email: info@nceft.org
http://www.nceft.org/index.html

NCEFT aims to improve the lives of children and adults with disabilities by providing equine-assisted therapy and equine-assisted activities and promoting research and education in the field of hippotherapy.

North American Riding for the Handicapped Association

PO Box 33150
Denver, CO 80233 USA
Phone: 303-452-1212; Toll-free: 800-369-7433
http://www.narha.org

Provides therapeutic riding for individuals with disabilities; offers training and certification for instructors working with the disabled; sponsors educational programs.

Paws With a Cause

4646 South Div.
Wayland, MI 49348
Phone: 800-253-7297
http://www.pawswithacause.org

Trains assistance dogs nationally for people with disabilities and provides lifetime team support that encourages independence; promotes awareness through education.

People-Animals-Love

4900 Massachusetts Ave. NW, Ste. 330
Washington, DC 20016 USA
Phone: 202-966-2171
http://www.peopleanimalslove.org

Founded in 1981 by a Washington, D.C.-area veterinarian, this volunteer organization has brought "affection and companionship to more than 8,000 people at 19 nursing homes, hospitals, mental health centers and PAL Club, creating more than 20,000 chances for snuggling close or walking briskly."

PAWS (Pets Are Wonderful Support)

645 Harrison St, Suite 100
San Francisco, CA 94107
Phone: 415-979-9550
Email: info@pawssf.org
http://www.pawssf.org

PAWS was founded in response to the HIV/AIDS epidemic in San Francisco. While serving at The San Francisco AIDS Foundation Food Bank in 1986, volunteers noticed that some clients were neglecting their own nutrition and feeding donated food to their animal companions instead. This concern inspired the volunteers to create a special food bank to carry pet food and supplies. In response to a large-scale demand, PAWS became an independent, nonprofit organization in October 1987.

Still a volunteer-based organization, PAWS "provides for the comprehensive needs of companion animals for low-income persons with disabling HIV/AIDS and other disabling illnesses and for senior citizens. By providing these essential support services, educating the larger community on the benefits of the human-animal bond, and advocating for the rights of disabled individuals to keep service animals, PAWS improves the health and well-being of disabled individuals and the animals in their lives."

Therapet Animal Assisted Therapy Foundation

P.O. Box 305
Troup, Texas 75789
http://www.therapet.org

Founded by an occupational therapist, this organization uses animals in healing and rehabilitating acute and chronically ill people. As of 2009, Therapet had 85 dogs, 3 cats, and 8 miniature horses working in East Texas and has established similar programs in Montana, Hawaii, New York, Florida, New Mexico, Arizona, Virginia, and Louisiana.

Therapy Dogs International

88 Bartley Rd.
Flanders, NJ 07836
Phone: 973-252-9800
http://www.tdi-dog.org

Founded in 1976, this volunteer organization is dedicated to regulating, testing, and registering therapy dogs and their volunteer handlers for the purpose of visiting nursing homes, hospitals, and other institutions where therapy dogs may be needed.

COLLEGE, UNIVERSITY, AND OTHER RESEARCH CENTERS ON THE ANIMAL-HUMAN BOND

Animals and Society Institute (ASI)

2512 Carpenter Road
Suite #201 A2
Ann Arbor, MI 48108-1188
Phone: 734-677-9240
General inquiries: info@animalsandsociety.org
http://www.animalsandsociety.org

The Animals and Society Institute is "an independent research and education organization dedicated to advancing the status of animals in public policy and promoting the study of human-animal relationships." The Animals and Society Institute's primary programs include these focus areas: *Human-Animal Studies*, a multidisciplinary academic field devoted to understanding more about humankind's complex relationship with animals. The ASI edits two academic journals devoted to the subject (*Society and Animals* and the *Journal of Applied Animal Welfare Science*) and works with academics and institutions nationwide to develop courses, minors programs and more.

The Animals' Platform, a blueprint that can be used at the local, state and national level to promote new and stricter animal protection legislation and policy. The Platform can be viewed or downloaded, and is available on DVD. *AniCare*, a multifaceted, direct-intervention program developed in 1999 to help stop the cycle of violence between animal cruelty and human abuse. There are separate programs for adult and juvenile offenders. The ASI publishes training manuals and conducts national workshops for mental health professionals, social workers, law enforcement agencies and others on the front lines of this important societal issue.

Colorado State University

Argus Institute
Colorado State University Veterinary Teaching Hospital
300 W. Drake Rd.
Fort Collins, CO 80523
Administration: 970-297-4143
http://www.argusinstitute.colostate.edu

The Institute was named after Odysseus' dog in Homer's *Odyssey*, a legendary canine who lovingly remembered his master despite a 20-year separation. Its mission is to strengthen veterinarian-client-patient communication and support relationships between people and their companion animals; offer support to people who are facing challenges surrounding their pet's healthcare; and provide community outreach through the student-run Pet Hospice Program and the Human-Animal Bond Club.

Purdue University

Center for the Human Animal-Bond
Purdue University School of Veterinary Medicine
625 Harrison Street. West Lafayette, IN 47907
Phone: 765-494-0854
http://www.vet.purdue.edu/chab/index.htm

Founded in 1982, the Center for Applied Ethology and Human-Animal Interaction studied these relationships and disseminated its findings to scientists and the public. In 1997, the name was changed to the Center for the Human-Animal Bond to reflect the relationship that exists between people and the animals that share this earth.

"The Center is committed to expanding our knowledge of the interrelationships between people, animals, and their environment. The Center is concerned with all aspects of human-animal interaction and welfare including companion, farmed domestic species, and wildlife. An emphasis is placed on humane ethics in managing our living resources."

Tufts University School of Veterinary Medicine

Tufts Center For Animals and Public Policy
200 Westboro Road
North Grafton, MA 01536
Phone: 508-839-7991
http://www.tufts.edu/vet/cfa

The Center for Animals and Public Policy was founded in 1983 at the Cummings School of Veterinary Medicine at Tufts University. The guiding vision was an institute for higher education and policy study that would investigate the scientific, ethical, legal,and social implications of human-animal relationships.

The Master of Science in Animals and Public Policy was established in 1995. Students in this intensive 12-month program explore human-animal relationships from an interdisciplinary perspective.

Tuskegee University

Center for the Study of Human-Animal Interdependent Relationships
1200 W. Montgomery Rd.
Tuskegee Inst, AL 36088
www.tuskegee.edu/bond

"The mission for the Center for the Study of Human-Animal Interdependent Relationships at Tuskegee University's School of Veterinary Medicine is to use a multidisciplinary approach to studying, strengthening, and promoting the health benefits that people and animals may derive from one another.

"Its mission is built on the belief that the interdependent relationships between people and animals is to be respected, valued, protected, and enhanced."

The Center was founded in 1997 and is funded in part by a grant under the Excellence in Minority Medical Education Program of the Health Resources and Service Administration (HRSA) of the U.S. Public Health Service.

University of California-Davis

Center for Companion Animal Health (CCAH)
School of Veterinary Medicine
University of California-Davis
One Shields Avenue
Davis, California 95616-8782
Phone 530-752-7295
http://www.vetmed.ucdavis.edu/CCAH

Founded in 1992, the Center for Companion Animal Health provides a core program in all aspects of health, well-being, and diseases of companion animals, which is administered by the faculty of both the UC-Davis Veterinary and Medical schools.

The mission is to improve the health of companion animals by providing financial support for academic studies on diseases affecting dogs, cats, and other small alternative pets. The CCAH also develops and supports programs that will benefit pets and their owners.

University of Minnesota

CENSHARE—Center to Study Human-Animal Relationships and Environments
717 Delaware St SE, Rm 130
Minneapolis, MN 55455-2040
phone 612-626-1975 or 612-625-7546
http://www.censhare.umn.edu/

The mission of CENSHARE is "to create opportunities to acquire, disseminate, and apply knowledge about the relationship between animals, humans, and their shared environment so that our informed choices improve the quality of life for all."

Established in 1981, this Center promotes the quality of life for people and animals through behavior research, educational opportunities, and a forum for public policy making.

University of Missouri

Research Center for Human-Animal Interaction (ReCHAI)
Clydesdale Annex #2
900 East Campus Drive
Columbia MO 65211
Email: rechai@missouri.edu
Phone: 573-882-2266
http://rechai.missouri.edu/links.htm

According to the organization's website, ReCHAI is designed to

- Develop a program for research and education to study the health benefits of human-animal interaction (HAI).
- Promote the science of HAI.
- Further the understanding and value of the relationship between humans and animals.
- Document evidence demonstrating Animal Assisted Activity (AAA) as a beneficial form of complementary therapy.
- Celebrate and better document the benefits of HAI.
- Foster educational and research opportunities for MU students.
- Collaborate with other centers nationally and internationally to promote HAI.
- Foster public understanding of benefits of HAI.

Some research projects (listed on website):

- "Pet Attachment, Health and Well-Being of Ethnic Elders" was a study to what extent ethnic elders are attached to their pets and whether pets are part of their fitness activities.
- "Walking for Healthy Hearts" is a study about what motivated residents of public housing to walk with a trained visitor dog.
- "Pet Pals" is a study of older adults who were newly relocated to a nursing home.
- "Owner Perceptions of Visits with their Hospitalized Pets" asked dog owners their perspective of visiting their dog while it was hospitalized in the ICU.
- "Ask the Community: Barriers & Facilitators to Exercise & Physical Activity" aims to identify existing exercise and physical activity resources in the community.
- "Walk a Hound, Lose a Pound and Stay Fit for Seniors" studies the effects of shelter dog walking on fitness and social support of older adults.

University of Pennsylvania

Center for the Interaction of Animals and Society (CIAS)
University of Pennsylvania School of Veterinary Medicine
3800 Spruce St.
Philadelphia, PA 19106
Phone: 215-898-5438
http://research.vet.upenn.edu/Default.aspx?alias=research.vet.upenn.edu/cias

According to the website:

The Center for the Interaction of Animals and Society (CIAS) is a multi-disciplinary research center within the School of Veterinary Medicine at the University of Pennsylvania. It was re-established in 1997 to provide a forum for addressing the many practical and moral issues arising from the interactions of animals and society. The study of human-animal interactions is still a new and developing field that straddles the boundaries between traditional academic disciplines. For this reason, the CIAS strives for an interdisciplinary approach and the involvement of scholars and researchers from a wide variety of different backgrounds and interests.

The broad goal of the CIAS is to promote understanding of human-animal interactions and relationships across a wide range of contexts including companion animals, farm animals, laboratory animals, zoo animals, and free-living wild animals. More specifically, the CIAS aims to:

1. Study the positive and negative influence of people's relationships with animals on their physical and mental health and well being.
2. Investigate the impact of these relationships on the behavior and welfare of the animals involved.
3. Encourage constructive, balanced, and well-informed debate and discussion on the ethics of animal use.
4. Use the knowledge and information gained from this work to benefit people, and promote the humane use and treatment of animals.

Virginia Commonwealth University

Center for Human-Animal Interaction (CHAI)
c/o Professor Sandra Barker
P.O. Box: 980710
Richmond, VA 23298-0565
E-mail: sbbarker@vcu.edu
Phone: 804-827-PAWS (7297)
http://www.medschool.vcu.edu/community/chai/index.html

Established in the VCU School of Medicine in June 2001, the purpose of the Center for Human-Animal Interaction is to provide a formal structure for and promote interdisciplinary and inter-institutional research, clinical practice, and educational activities related to the human-animal relationship. Housed within the Department of Psychiatry in the VCU School of Medicine, CHAI is the only center of its kind based in a medical school.

To achieve its mission, the research goal is to increase knowledge of the benefits of the human-animal interaction through interdisciplinary research; the clinical goal is to enhance health and well being through animal-assisted therapy and pet visitation. Volunteers are required to maintain their volunteer status by participating in annual reorientation, annual health screening and in any other activities required by VCUHS; the educational goal is to improve understanding of the benefits of the human-animal interaction. The Center for Human-Animal Interaction offers a number of programs and services.

Washington State University

People-Pet Partnership
College of Veterinary Medicine
P. O. Box 647010
Washington State University
Pullman, WA 99164-7010
Phone: 509-335-7347

The Pet-People Partnership (PPP), a public service program in the Center for the Study of Animal Well-Being (CSAW) in the College of Veterinary

Medicine, "was created to more fully understand the human–animal bond and to promote the humane treatment of companion animals."

Through education, research, and outreach, the PPP provides a number of important public services, including:

Palouse Area Therapeutic Horsemanship (PATH): A program that provides recreational therapeutic horseback riding to people with emotional, mental, and physical disabilities.

Human-Animal Bond Research: Our research seeks to better understand the significant bond between animals and humans, how caring for animals enhances human well-being, and how the bond between animals and humans influences veterinary medicine.

Pet Education Partnership: An online curriculum to teach children responsible pet ownership.

Primary Documents

Since this reference book tries to cover an enormous amount of information in only one volume, many of the following documents are included to supplement or expand upon the narrative text and/or bibliography. Other documents are included because even though they don't address matters directly related to the commonly accepted definition of animal-assisted therapy, they focus on major forms of animal care for human companions or other aspects of the human-animal bond.

The first report, "CommonlyAsked Questions about Service Animals in Places of Business," fits into the latter category. From a legal perspective, service animals are considered different from therapy animals. According to the 1990 Americans with Disabilities Act (ADA), a dog is considered a "service dog" if it has been "individually trained to do work or perform tasks for the benefit of a person with a disability." Thus, service animals are defined by federal law and they and their human companions are granted legal rights in businesses and public accommodations. Therapy animals, by contrast, are not specifically protected under such federal legal provisions, but many states do explicitly allow these animals to visit long-term health care facilities, except in places that have "no pets" policies. These therapy animals are usually the personal pets of their handlers and work with them to provide physical and emotional services to institutionalized individuals and others.

Issued by the Disability Rights Section of the U.S. Department of Justice, this first document ("Commonly Asked Questions") includes questions and answers for business owners who need to know the

ADA requirements for providing access to service animals who accompany people with disabilities. The Assistance Dogs International has established minimum standards for training "hearing" dogs, as listed in the second document (Document #2).

The next set reprints guidelines and other types of information published on the Web sites of various professional and animal-assisted therapy organizations. The American Veterinary Medical Association—the pre-eminent U.S. organization of veterinarians working in private and corporate practice, government, industry, academia, and uniformed services—has published guidelines (Documents #3 and #4) for animal-assisted activity, animal-assisted therapy, and resident animal programs.

The next set of documents was compiled by the Utah-based group Intermountain Therapy Animals, a decade-old organization that has pioneered the use of dogs in schools and libraries to assist children with reading difficulties. (Please see Chapter 2, Programs for Children, for more detailed information). Their Web site provides the following reprinted documents: FAQs on their innovative R.E.A.D. program, which uses therapy dogs to sit beside children with reading problems as they read aloud (Document #5); a pet suitability for therapy service index that discusses the qualities needed by both the companion animal and its human handler (Document #6;) and guidelines for trainers of therapy animals (Document #7)

Many people who are unfamiliar with service or therapy animals do not know the proper way to behave in their presence so Canine Companions for Independence has published a helpful list of guidelines for such occasions (Document #8).

Although this book focuses almost exclusively on animal-assisted therapy in the United States (with very brief mentions of Canada), the concluding documents offer some important and little-known information about the use of this type of therapy outside the United States. The first document (Document #9) contains the Code of Ethics of the Israeli Association of Animal-Assisted Psychotherapy. The next article (Document #10) was authored by Italian scientists and therapists and provides an analysis of the beneficial effects of both animal-assisted therapy and animal-assisted activities in some parts of Italy. Finally, although the Controversies chapter briefly discusses some ethical issues arising out of this therapy, a much deeper and more philosophically rigorous discussion of AAT can be found in *The Moral Basis of Animal-Assisted Therapy* published in the journal *Anthrozoos* (Document #11). Written by Tzachi Zamir, an Israeli social philosopher, this lengthy and well-argued essay raises important issues about the therapy and its use of different types of animals.

Document 1: Commonly Asked Questions about Service Animals in Places of Business

> Source: U.S. Department of Justice; Civil Rights Division. "COMMONLY ASKED QUESTIONS ABOUT SERVICE ANIMALS IN PLACES OF BUSINESS." http://www.ada.gov/qasrvc.htm (accessed July 1, 2010).

1. Q: What are the laws that apply to my business?

A: Under the Americans with Disabilities Act (ADA), privately owned businesses that serve the public, such as restaurants, hotels, retail stores, taxicabs, theaters, concert halls, and sports facilities, are prohibited from discriminating against individuals with disabilities. The ADA requires these businesses to allow people with disabilities to bring their service animals onto business premises in whatever areas customers are generally allowed.

2. Q: What is a service animal?

A: The ADA defines a service animal as *any* guide dog, signal dog, or other animal individually trained to provide assistance to an individual with a disability. If they meet this definition, animals are considered service animals under the ADA regardless of whether they have been licensed or certified by a state or local government.

Service animals perform some of the functions and tasks that the individual with a disability cannot perform for him or herself. Guide dogs are one type of service animal, used by some individuals who are blind. This is the type of service animal with which most people are familiar. But there are service animals that assist persons with other kinds of disabilities in their day-to-day activities. Some examples include:

- Alerting persons with hearing impairments to sounds.
- Pulling wheelchairs or carrying and picking up things for persons with mobility impairments.
- Assisting persons with mobility impairments with balance.
- A service animal is *not* a pet.

3. Q: How can I tell if an animal is really a service animal and not just a pet?

A: Some, but not all, service animals wear special collars and harnesses. Some, but not all, are licensed or certified and have identification papers. If you are not certain that an animal is a service animal, you may ask the person who has the animal if it is a service animal required because of a disability. However, an individual who is going to a restaurant or theater is not likely to be carrying documentation of his or her medical condition or disability. Therefore, such documentation generally may not be required as a condition for providing service to an individual accompanied by a service animal. Although a number of states have programs to certify service animals, you may not insist on proof of state certification before permitting the service animal to accompany the person with a disability.

4. Q: What must I do when an individual with a service animal comes to my business?
A: The service animal must be permitted to accompany the individual with a disability to all areas of the facility where customers are normally allowed to go. An individual with a service animal may not be segregated from other customers.

5. Q: I have always had a clearly posted "no pets" policy at my establishment. Do I still have to allow service animals in?
A: Yes. A service animal is *not* a pet. The ADA requires you to modify your "no pets" policy to allow the use of a service animal by a person with a disability. This does not mean you must abandon your "no pets" policy altogether but simply that you must make an exception to your general rule for service animals.

6. Q: My county health department has told me that *only* a guide dog has to be admitted. If I follow those regulations, am I violating the ADA?
A: Yes, if you refuse to admit any other type of service animal on the basis of local health department regulations or other state or local laws. The ADA provides greater protection for individuals with disabilities and so it takes priority over the local or state laws or regulations.

7. Q: Can I charge maintenance or cleaning fee for customers who bring service animals into my business?
A: No. Neither a deposit nor a surcharge may be imposed on an individual with a disability as a condition to allowing a service animal to accompany the individual with a disability, even if deposits are routinely required for pets. However, a public accommodation may charge its customers with disabilities if a service animal causes damage so long as it is the regular practice of the entity to charge non-disabled customers for the same types of damages. For example, a hotel can charge a guest with a disability for the cost of repairing or cleaning furniture damaged by a service animal if it is the hotel's policy to charge when non-disabled guests cause such damage.

8. Q: I operate a private taxicab and I don't want animals in my taxi; they smell, shed hair, and sometimes have "accidents." Am I violating the ADA if I refuse to pick up someone with a service animal?
A: Yes. Taxicab companies may not refuse to provide services to individuals with disabilities. Private taxicab companies are also prohibited from

charging higher fares or fees for transporting individuals with disabilities and their service animals than they charge to other persons for the same or equivalent service.

9. Q: Am I responsible for the animal while the person with a disability is in my business?
A: No. The care or supervision of a service animal is solely the responsibility of his or her owner. You are not required to provide care or food or a special location for the animal.

10. Q: What if a service animal barks or growls at other people or otherwise acts out of control?
A: You may exclude any animal, including a service animal, from your facility when that animal's behavior poses a direct threat to the health or safety of others. For example, any service animal that displays vicious behavior towards other guests or customers may be excluded. You may not make assumptions, however, about how a particular animal is likely to behave based on your past experience with other animals. Each situation must be considered individually.

Although a public accommodation may exclude any service animal that is out of control, it should give the individual with a disability who uses the service animal the option of continuing to enjoy its goods and services without having the service animal on the premises.

11. Q: Can I exclude an animal that doesn't really seem dangerous but is disruptive to my business?
A: There may be a few circumstances when a public accommodation is not required to accommodate a service animal—that is, when doing so would result in a fundamental alteration to the nature of the business. Generally, this is not likely to occur in restaurants, hotels, retail stores, theaters, concert halls, and sports facilities. But when it does, for example, when a dog barks during a movie, the animal can be excluded.

If you have further questions about service animals or other requirements of the ADA, you may call the U.S. Department of Justice's toll-free ADA Information Line at 800-514-0301 (voice) or 800-514-0383 (TDD).

DOCUMENT 2: MINIMUM STANDARDS FOR TRAINING HEARING DOGS (ADI)

Assistance Dogs International, Inc. "Minimum Standard for Training Hearing Dogs." http://www.assistancedogsinternational.org/Standards/HearingDogStandards.php (accessed July 1, 2010). Copyright © 1997–2010, Assistance Dogs International, Inc. All rights reserved. Used by permission.

These are intended to be minimum standards for all assistance dog programs that are members or provisional members with ADI. All programs are encouraged to work at levels above the minimums.

1. The hearing dog must respond to basic obedience commands from the handler 90% of the time on the first ask in all public and home environments. The dog must respond to the trained sound with an alerting behavior within 15 seconds from the beginning of the sound.
2. The hearing dog should demonstrate basic obedience skills by responding to voice and/or hand signals for sitting, staying in place, lying down, walking in a controlled position near the client, and coming to the client when called.
3. The hearing dog must meet all of the standards as laid out in the ADI Minimum Standards for Dogs in Public and should be equally well behaved in the home environment.
4. Sound Awareness Skills. Upon hearing a sound, the hearing dog should alert the client by making physical contact or by some other behavior, so the client is aware when a trained sound occurs. The dog should then specifically indicate or lead the person to the source of the sound. All dogs must be trained to alert the handler to at least three (3) sounds.
5. The client must be provided with enough instruction to be able to meet the ADI Minimum Standards for Assistance Dogs in Public. Clients must be able to demonstrate:
   • That their dog can alert to three (3) different sounds.
   • Knowledge of acceptable training techniques.
   • An understanding of canine care and health.
   • The ability to continue to train, problem solve, and add new skills with their hearing dog.
   • Knowledge of local access laws and appropriate public behavior.

   The program must document monthly follow ups with clients for the first 6 months following placement. Personal contact will be done by qualified staff or program volunteers within 12 months of graduation and annually thereafter.

   Identification of the hearing dog will be accomplished with the laminated ID card with a photo (s) and names of the dog and partner. In public the dog must wear a cape, harness, backpack, or other similar piece of equipment or clothing with a logo that is clear and easy to read and identifiable as an assistance dog.

   The program staff must demonstrate the knowledge of deafness, deaf culture, and hearing impairment. A staff member or agent must know basic sign language. The program shall make available to staff and volunteers educational material on deafness, deaf culture and hearing impairment.

   The client must abide by the ADI Minimum Standards of Assistance Dog Partners.

Prior to placement the hearing dog must meet the ADI Standards and Ethics Regarding Dogs, be spayed/neutered and have current vaccination certificates as determined by their veterinarian and applicable laws. It is the program's responsibility to inform the client of any special health or maintenance care requirements for each dog.

DOCUMENT 3: GUIDELINES FOR ANIMAL-ASSISTED ACTIVITY, ANIMAL-ASSISTED THERAPY, AND RESIDENTIAL ANIMAL PROGRAMS)

American Veterinary Medical Association. "Guidelines of Animal-Assisted Activity and Therapy Programs." http://www.avma.org/products/hab/therapy.pdf (accessed July 1, 2010). Copyright © 2007, American Veterinary Medical Association. All rights reserved. Used by permission.

Statement of Policy

When the AVMA officially recognized, in 1982, that the human-animal bond was important to client and community health, it acknowledged that the human-animal bond has existed for thousands of years and that this relationship has major importance for veterinary medicine. As veterinary medicine serves society, it fulfills human and animal needs. Animal-assisted activities, animal-assisted therapy, and resident animal programs are included and endorsed by human healthcare providers as cost-effective interventions for specific patient populations in various acute and rehabilitative care facilities. Veterinarians, as individuals and professionals, are uniquely qualified to provide community service via such programs and to aid in scientific evaluation and documentation of the health benefits of the human-animal bond. Animal-assisted activities, animal-assisted therapy, and resident animal programs should be governed by basic standards, be regularly monitored, and be staffed by appropriately trained personnel. The health and welfare of the humans and animals involved must be ensured. Veterinarians' involvement in these programs from their inception is critical because they serve as advocates for the health and welfare of animals participating in these programs, and as experts in zoonotic disease transmission.

Definitions[1]

Animal-assisted activities (AAA) provide opportunities for motivation, education, or recreation to enhance quality of life. Animal-assisted activities are delivered in a variety of environments by specially trained professionals, paraprofessionals, or volunteers in association with animals that meet specific criteria.

Animal-assisted therapy (AAT) is a goal-directed intervention in which an animal meeting specific criteria is an integral part of the treatment process. Animal-assisted therapy is delivered and/or directed by health or human service providers working within the scope of their profession.

Animal-assisted therapy is designed to promote improvement in human physical, social, emotional, or cognitive function. Animal-assisted therapy is provided in a variety of settings, and may be group or individual in nature. The process is documented and evaluated.

Resident animals (RA) live in a facility full time, are owned by the facility, and are cared for by staff, volunteers, and residents. Some RA may be formally included in facility activity and therapy schedules after proper screening and training. Others may participate in spontaneous or planned interactions with facility residents and staff.

Human-animal support services (HASS) enhance and encourage responsible and humane interrelationships of people, animals, and nature.

Benefits of AAA, AAT, and RA Programs

Interactions with animals can provide emotional and physical health benefits for diverse human populations, including the elderly, children, physically handicapped, deaf, blind, emotionally or physically ill, and the incarcerated. By serving as communication catalysts among residents, healthcare staff, and visitors, animals can socialize healthcare facilities. They also may serve as diversions during anxiety-provoking procedures, such as physical examinations. With proper training, animals can be taught to reinforce rehabilitative behaviors in patients, such as throwing a ball, walking, or verbal responses. Hippotherapy (therapeutic horseback riding) has been reported to improve posture, balance, and coordination. Sense barriers may interfere with human-human interactions and tend to isolate affected individuals; however, verbal communication and sight are not necessary for positive interactions with animals and these interactions may facilitate communication with human handlers or healthcare providers. Animals can be included in behavior modification programs as a source of support and diversion during threatening situations, such as counseling. Some therapists have suggested that animals provide a type of reality therapy (by empathizing with the animal's natural instincts, patients see their own life more objectively). The training of animals provides troubled adolescents and the incarcerated with goals and an object of contact comfort.

Residential pets provide opportunities for physical activity or rehabilitation through their need for routine care, such as the construction of habitats, feeding, grooming, and exercise. The responsibility of caring for animals may also provide residents with a sense of purpose and a perceived need to take better care of them.

Concerns Related to AAA, AAT, and RA Programs

Occasionally program participants become so involved with the animals that they become possessive of those animals and an atmosphere of competition rather than social cooperation develops. Patients may perceive that an animal has rejected them, usually because of unrealistic expectations of the animal's behavior toward them, and this can exacerbate low self-esteem. Death of an animal may generate intense feelings of grief and sometimes guilt in patients and staff. Human injury may result because of inappropriate animal selection, handling, or lack of supervision; likewise, animals may be abused or accidentally injured. Zoonotic diseases may be transmitted if careful veterinary supervision and sound sanitation practices are not an integral part of the AAA, AAT, or RA program, and participants' potential allergic reactions to animal dander are always a concern.

Veterinary Involvement

No one is better able to monitor the health and welfare of animals involved in AAA, AAT, and RA programs than a veterinarian. Veterinarians can provide answers to fundamental questions concerning animal husbandry, health, handling, and behavior, and they are the recognized experts in zoonotic disease.

Veterinarians may become active participants in AAA, AAT, and RA programs after being approached by a client, or the director of a healthcare or human service facility for assistance. Veterinarians may also initiate such programs as cooperative projects between human and animal healthcare providers and agencies.

Key Components for Successful Use of Animals in AAA, AAT, and RA Programs[2]

Interdisciplinary cooperation—Successful AAA, AAT, and RA programs are inherently interdisciplinary and present a wonderful opportunity for veterinarians, physicians, nursing staff, activity directors, therapists, and volunteers to work together toward a common goal.

Planning—Establish realistic goals and expectations. Anticipation of possible problems and development of solutions prior to their occurrence can avoid conflicts that cause program failure.

Supervision—Staff and administrative supervision of AAT, AAT, and RA programs are required to protect the welfare of human and animal participants. All personnel need to be made aware that the program is in place and that it is considered to play an integral role in patient care. If an animal becomes a permanent resident of a facility, one individual should be assigned primary responsibility for its care and management, including arrangements for weekend and holiday care.

Animal selection—Animals should be selected on the basis of type, breed, size, age, sex, and, particularly, natural behavior appropriate for the intended use. Only animals with known medical and behavioral histories should be used, and medical and behavioral assessments should be performed prior to placing animals in a program. Animals should have been, and should be, trained by use of positive reinforcement. Animals must be chosen with the target population in mind. A boisterous, overactive dog may be friendly, but inappropriate for a nursing home in which many patients are using walkers. A visiting calf or lamb may be more effective with patients who have rural backgrounds than would a caged rodent.

Animal health, human health, and environmental concerns—A wellness program should be instituted for animals participating in AAA, AAT, and RA programs to prevent or minimize human exposure to common zoonotic diseases such as rabies, psittacosis, salmonellosis, toxoplasmosis, campylobacteriosis, and giardiasis. Need for specific screening tests should be cooperatively determined by the program's attending veterinarian(s) and physician(s). Animals should also be appropriately immunized and licensed. With respect to immunization for rabies, the current Compendium of Animal Rabies Prevention and Control (prepared by the National Association of State Public Health Veterinarians and published annually in the Journal of the American Veterinary Medical Association) and/or state guidelines should be followed. If the animal is to reside at a facility, provisions must be made for its feeding, watering, housing, grooming, and exercise. Associated noise and waste disposal problems must also be solved.

Human-animal interactions and welfare—During interactive sessions, the welfare of residents, animals, volunteers, staff, and visitors must be considered. Introductions of animals and human participants must be arranged and supervised, because some individuals may not enjoy interacting with animals or may have physical or emotional problems that contraindicate such interactions. Animals should be an integral part of a treatment program and not a reward for appropriate behavior on the part of the human participant. Animals should be monitored closely for clinical signs of stress and should have ample opportunity and space for solitude. Any problems or incidents that occur must be reported to appropriate supervisory staff.

Laws Governing AAA, AAT, and RA Programs

Most states allow animals in long-term healthcare facilities and other institutions, with some restrictions. Animals are usually not allowed in food preparation and serving rooms or in areas where sterile conditions are maintained. Health certificates for animals may be required. Program organizers should check with state and local officials for specific regulations.

Liability

Most institutions should be able to include an AAA, AAT, or RA program as one of their operational programs without additional insurance riders. Individuals providing AAA, AAT, or RA programs for these institutions should be able to obtain protection for their work under their existing individual or agency personal insurance policy. They may also be covered under the institution's insurance policy as a welcomed visitor. In all cases, the institution, agency, therapist, or volunteer should consult their respective insurance agents to ensure adequate protection.

Getting Started

An AAA, AAT, or RA program should be implemented only after there has been adequate advance preparation and discussion by everyone involved. Program organizers should be familiar with AAA, AAT, or RA concepts, available animal certification methods and programs, and national, state, and local laws pertaining to use of animals in facilities. Good communication among all individuals involved is essential. Roles of participants must be clearly defined and basic standards must be established to protect human and animal health, ensure the safety of participants, manage associated risks, and appropriately allocate program resources.[3] Workload for program and facility staff must be appropriately and carefully managed, and adequate training must be provided. Participants must understand and respect principles of confidentiality. All AAA, AAT, and RA programs should include a veterinarian as a key participant so the health and welfare of humans and animals involved are protected.

Checklist

1. Assess the need for an AAA, AAT, or/RA program. Will it augment, and can it be readily incorporated into, existing treatment programs?
2. Establish realistic and measurable goals and objectives. Evaluate staff, facility, and financial resources to ensure that implementation is feasible.
3. Gain acceptance for your program by explaining its potential to key administrators and enlisting their assistance during development of protocols.
4. Determine what animals will best serve the needs of program participants. Consider the population to be served and any physical and psychological limitations. Become familiar with existing health department regulations concerning animals in facilities, because certain animals may be prohibited. If animals are to be resident, their husbandry must be addressed.

5. Develop protocols and training programs for staff, volunteers, and animals.
6. Assess zoonotic disease risks and develop appropriate procedures for minimizing those risks.
7. Measure the successes and failures of your program through medical record charting, case studies, questionnaires, videotapes, or formal research.

Notes

1. Definitions Development Task Force of the Standards Committee. Generic terms and definitions. Handbook for animal-assisted activities and animal-assisted therapy. Renton, WA: Delta Society; 1992, 48.

2. Arkow P. How to start a "pet therapy" program: a guidebook for health care professionals. Colorado Springs, CO: The Humane Society of the Pikes Peak Region; 1998.

3. International Association of Human-Animal Interaction Organizations. The IAHAIO Prague guidelines on animal-assisted activities and animal-assisted therapy. Renton, WA: Delta Society; 1998.

Suggested Reading

Arkow P. Animal-assisted therapy and activities: a study resource guide and bibliography for the use of companion animals in selected therapies. Stratford, NJ (self-published but available through some bookstores and online book services); 2004.

American Veterinary Medical Association. Wellness guidelines for animals in animal-assisted activity, animal-assisted therapy, and resident animal programs. www.avma.org/issues/policy/animal_assisted_activity.asp.

Burch MR, Bustad LK, Duncan SL, et al. The role of pets in therapeutic programmes. In: Robinson I, ed. The Waltham book of human-animal interaction: benefits and responsibilities of pet ownership. Tarrytown, NY: Elsevier Science Inc; 1995:55–69.

Delta Society. Standards of practice for animal-assisted activities and therapy. Renton, WA: Delta Society; 1999.

Fine A, ed. Handbook on animal-assisted therapy: theoretical foundations and guidelines for practice. San Diego, CA: Academic Press; 2006.

Other Resources

For the most current information on zoonotic diseases, contact the American Veterinary Medical Association, 1931 North Meacham Road, Suite 100, Schaumburg, Illinois 60173 (www.avma.org), or the Centers for Disease Control and Prevention, 1600 Clifton Road, NE, Atlanta, GA 30333 (www.cdc.gov).

DOCUMENT 4: WELLNESS GUIDELINES FOR ANIMALS IN ANIMAL-ASSISTED ACTIVITY, ANIMAL-ASSISTED THERAPY, AND RESIDENT ANIMAL PROGRAMS

American Veterinary Medical Association. "Wellness Guidelines For Animal-Assisted Activity, Animal-Assisted Therapy, Resident Animal

Active or passive interactions with animals can be of great psychosocial and physical benefit for populations with special needs. Veterinarians who wish to be involved in human-animal interaction activities and programs must prepare themselves to play a vital role. These guidelines are designed for veterinarians just entering this exciting field, as well as those who may have experience enabling these services in their communities. Participating veterinarians will be presented with challenges and questions requiring investigation, and often further education, before appropriate decisions can be made. Some of the most common concerns facing veterinarians involved in animal-assisted activity (AAA), animal-assisted therapy (AAT), and resident animal (RA) programs are zoonotic disease risks and behavioral problems. These guidelines are not intended to address these complex issues in detail. Instead, they were developed to provide veterinarians with a platform on which to build a knowledge base, to help ensure that the animals involved are protected, and to maximize the therapeutic applications of the human-animal bond. Veterinarians should use the concepts presented here as a starting point and build on them by consulting other authoritative resources.

Definitions

Animal-assisted activities (AAA)[1]—Animal-assisted activities provide opportunities for motivation, education, or recreation to enhance quality of life. Animal-assisted activities are delivered in various environments by specially trained professionals, paraprofessionals, and volunteers in association with animals that meet specific criteria. Included are "meet and greet" activities that involve pets and their handlers visiting people on a scheduled or spontaneous basis, as well as programs permitting family members or friends of facility residents to bring their own pet or the resident's pet for a visit. The same activity may be repeated with many individuals or be conducted in groups; unlike therapy programs, they are not tailored to a particular person or medical condition. Visit content is spontaneous and visits are as long or as short as necessary.

Animal-assisted therapy (AAT)—Animal-assisted therapy is a goal-directed intervention in which an animal that meets specific criteria is an integral part of the treatment process. These programs are usually directed and delivered by human health or human services professionals with specialized expertise and within the scope of practice of their profession. Animal-assisted therapy is designed to improve human physical, social, emotional, and cognitive (e.g., thinking and intellectual skills) function and animals may be formally included in activities such as physical, occupational, or speech therapy. Therapy programs are provided in a variety of settings and may involve individuals or groups. In AAT, specified goals and objectives are determined for each patient and their progress is evaluated and documented.

Resident animals (RA)—Resident animals live in a facility full time, are owned by the facility, and are cared for by staff, volunteers, and residents. Some RA may be formally included in facility activity and therapy schedules after proper screening and training. Others may participate in spontaneous or planned interactions with facility residents and staff.

Responsible person (RP)—At least one person must be responsible for the health, behavior, and welfare of the animal(s) involved in these programs on a daily basis. This individual is critically important to the wellness and welfare of the animal. In some instances, the RP will be an owner or a handler. In the case of RA, the RP may be one or more staff members to whom these responsibilities have been specifically assigned.

Guiding Principles and Dynamics

Wellness programs should be designed to provide reasonable assurance that animals used in AAA, AAT, and RA programs are (1) healthy, so as to reduce the bi-directional risk of transmission of zoonoses; (2) behaviorally appropriate for the program, and (3) protected from being harmed by participation in the program. A wellness program goes beyond annual physical examinations and associated vaccinations and medications. Rather, it involves continuous monitoring by the RP and periodic monitoring by the veterinarian for the purpose of developing preventive care strategies that will enhance the health and welfare of the animal. Total wellness encompasses the physical and behavioral attributes of the animal, as well as the characteristics of interaction between people and animals participating in the program.

Specifically,

- To ensure the welfare of human and animal participants, a veterinarian should be actively involved in all AAA, AAT, and RA programs. Positive human and animal outcomes are dependent on a close partnership and frequent communication between the veterinarian and the RP, as well as good communication with licensed therapists (e.g., occupational and physical therapists) and a qualified animal behaviorist.
- The attending veterinarian should be familiar with the types of tasks that will be expected of the animal(s) and have experience with the physical and behavioral characteristics of the species to be used in the program. This is particularly important when physical or behavioral changes are detected in animals, because this information,

in addition to good communication between the veterinarian and the RP, will help the veterinarian assess whether changes are caused by participation in the AAA, AAT, or RA program.

- A mechanism should be in place to permit the veterinarian to periodically assess the physical and behavioral health and welfare of the animal(s) involved. The wellness program should proactively enhance the health and welfare of the animal(s) and should include regularly scheduled examinations and preventive care.

- Wellness programs should be tailored to fit the needs of individual animals. Species, age, breed, and any risk factors that could jeopardize an animal's health and welfare should be considered. Dogs and cats should not be used in these programs until they are at least six months old and are prepared for participation, and the special needs of elderly animals should be addressed. Appropriate ages for other species should also be considered, taking into account physical and zoonotic risks, behavioral appropriateness, and stressors that may adversely affect young or elderly animals in these programs.

- Access to veterinary care must be available as needed between scheduled appointments.

- Wellness programs should include regular vaccination; parasite prevention and control; selected screening for common diseases and conditions; behavioral evaluation; preventive medical, dental, nutritional, and behavioral care, including environmental enrichment; and an assessment of genetic health when appropriate.

- A decline in animal wellness may manifest itself as a physical or behavioral change. Because wellness is dynamic, wellness programs should be flexible and modified to accommodate the changing needs of animals as they age or as a result of participation in AAA, AAT, or RA programs.

- The RP must be willing to share the results of an animal's medical and behavioral evaluations (usually in summary format) with regulatory agencies that have legal oversight for the target populations of AAA, AAT, and RA programs.

- Daily recommendations concerning animal wellness must be readily available to all members of a household or facility so that everyone can be involved in maintaining the health and welfare of animal(s) involved in AAA, AAT, and RA programs. However, sharing recommendations and encouraging others to promote animal wellness does not eliminate the need for, or duties of, a RP.

Selected Preventive Medical Strategies

- Wellness visits should include a thorough physical examination that includes assessment of nutritional and oral health, screening for selected infectious and parasitic diseases, evaluation of behavior and lifestyle factors related to the animal and others in the household or facility, a reproductive health assessment, and an evaluation for congenital diseases and/or conditions. Preexisting medical conditions or potential behavior problems that might be worsened by AAA, AAT, or RA activities should be documented and the RP informed about associated risks and medical or behavioral changes that might indicate worsening of the condition.

- Animals should be vaccinated for rabies (if appropriate for that species) in accordance with local and state ordinances or regulations. Other vaccinations should be given at appropriate intervals, as determined by the veterinarian, to be in the best interest of the animal, its RP, and the individuals with whom the animal will be in contact.

- Internal and external parasite prevention and control programs should be implemented in accordance with local risks and the life stage of the animal. The practitioner should keep in mind that these animals may not be candidates for certain topical insecticides because of the degree of handling and petting associated with AAA, AAT, and RA programs.

- Disabilities should not necessarily eliminate an animal from participation in AAA, AAT, or RA programs. Amputees or deaf animals, if otherwise healthy, can have a positive impact on special populations, providing their activities do not exacerbate their disabilities and that the ability that is lacking is not necessary for safe and effective interaction with the target population. Participation of animals having conditions that may affect their mobility should be evaluated in light of the physical facilities of the AAA, AAT, or RA program (e.g., a dog with hip dysplasia may have difficulty maneuvering stairs or long hallways). Disabled animals must be monitored closely by the RP and the attending veterinarian to ensure that the animal's participation does not exacerbate an existing medical condition or adversely affect its ability to provide needed services.

- Screening tests should be selected on the basis of their ability to identify medical problems in these animals and to reduce bi-directional risks of transmission of potential pathogens between animals and humans. Results of screening tests should be evaluated with regard to realistic risks to humans and animals. Appropriate treatment and risk management should be instituted if needed. Interactions of animals with immunocompromised individuals may justify use of certain screening tests that would not be necessary if those animals were only interacting with immunocompetent populations.

- The RP should be provided with information on maintaining the animal's hair coat and nail quality, and should be taught to do a basic assessment of their animal¡ls skin condition. Excessive grooming or bathing (including the use of harsh products) in preparation for AAA or AAT or as part of a maintenance protocol for a RA may be deleterious.

- Recommendations for health maintenance should include behavior management, daily exercise, play, diet, preventive dental care, and the potential advantages of spaying/neutering in selected species.
- Medications administered to participating animals should be reviewed for their appropriateness (e.g., animals treated with immunosuppressive medications may be at greater risk of contracting infectious agents).

Selected Preventive Behavioral Strategies

- During wellness visits, the attending veterinarian should specifically address behavioral health. Questions about the appropriateness or inappropriateness of elimination can reveal information that may relate to other training and health issues. Reports of inappropriate elimination should be probed to determine their possible association with participation in AAA, AAT, or RA programs. Behavioral changes may occur more frequently as animals age or if medical conditions cause discomfort or pain.
- Behaviors that could be considered inappropriate must be assessed in the context of RP expectations and tolerances. For example, some RP expect dogs to chew and cats to scratch. Behaviors tolerated in the home may not be acceptable in hospital or long-term care facilities and the RP should be counseled to this effect.
- Behaviors should be evaluated in the context of the general physical and behavioral health of the animal, as well as with respect to the animal's age and any preexisting conditions. For example, aggression may be a consequence of irritability associated with a medical condition. Changes in elimination frequency or volume may be associated with an underlying medical cause or be an effect of aging.
- The RP must ensure that resident animals are provided regular opportunities for play, quiet time, and rest separate from activities involving contacts with residents and staff. Similar consideration must be afforded animals used for AAA and AAT.
- The RP and facility residents should be educated about behavioral signs that might indicate that an animal is not enjoying an activity associated with AAA, AAT, or its residence in the facility. The RP and residents must carefully observe the animal's body language to detect signs of stress, discomfort, anxiety, or fear. They must also be aware of changes in sleep and eating patterns that could reflect excess stress or lack of proper care associated with the AAA, AAT, or RA program. The appearance of such signs should be discussed with a veterinarian to determine appropriate interventions. Interventions could include more frequent breaks, a "vacation" for

the animal, or discontinuing its participation depending on the factors associated with stress.

- Intervention options may need to be explored with a person knowledgeable in animal behavior and the operation of AAA, AAT, and RA programs to determine what is reasonable.

Other Considerations

- Animals should be trained not to pick things off the floor unless instructed by the RP. In some facilities, powerful human medications may accidentally fall to the floor or be intentionally offered to these animals.
- There should be a coding system to alert the RP to rooms that should not be entered because their occupants do not want to interact with animals or because of a greater risk of contracting or transmitting an infectious disease.
- The RP, veterinarian, and other involved parties must be aware that working animals may need to be retired because of their age, reduced enthusiasm for their job, or physical or behavioral concerns.

Note

1. Definitions Development Task Force of the Standards Committee. Generic Terms and Definitions. Handbook for animal-assisted activities and animal-assisted therapy. Renton, WA: Delta Society, 1992; 48.

Selected Resources

American Veterinary Medical Association. Guidelines for animal-assisted activity and therapy programs. Available online at www.avma.org/issues/policy/animal_assisted_guidelines.asp.

Bernard S. Animal-assisted therapy: a guide for health care professionals and volunteers. Whitehouse, Tex: Therapet, 1995.

Blanchard S. Companion parrot handbook: using nurturing guidance to create the best companion parrot possible. Alameda, Calif.: Pet Bird Information Council (PBIC), Inc., 1999.

Burch MR. Volunteering with your pet: how to get involved in animal-assisted therapy with any kind of pet. New York: Hungry Minds, Inc., 1996.

Center to Study Human-Animal Relationships and Environments (CENSHARE), University of Minnesota (www.censhare.umn.edu). Live-in animals videotape series (live-in dogs, cats, birds, fish, and rabbits).

Delta Society. Standards of practice for animal-assisted activities and therapy. Renton, Wash: Delta Society, 1999.

Fine A, ed., Handbook on animal-assisted therapy: theoretical foundations and guidelines for practice. San Diego, Calif: Academic Press, 2006.

Hart BL, Hart LA, eds. The pet connection: its influence on our health and quality of life. Minneapolis, Minn: University of Minnesota, 1984; 387–398.

McCulloch MJ. Pets in therapeutic programs for the aged. In: Anderson RK.

Nebbe LL. Nature as a guide: nature in counseling, therapy, and education. Minneapolis, Minn: Educational Media Corporation, 1995.

Thompson S. Wellness guidelines. Convention notes: American Veterinary Medical Association 136th Annual Convention. Schaumburg, Ill: American Veterinary Medical Association, 1999; 391–405.

Wilson CC, Turner DC, eds. Companion animals in human health. London, UK: Sage Publications, 1998.

DOCUMENT 5: F.A.Q.—R.E.A.D INDEX

Intermountain Therapy Animals. "Frequently Asked Questions About Reading Education Assistance Dogs (R.E.A.D.®)." http://www .therapyanimals.org/R.E.A.D.-Program.html (accessed July 1, 2010). Copyright © 1996-2009 by Intermountain Therapy Animals. All rights reserved. Reprinted by permission of Intermountain Therapy Animals.

Please tell me about the R.E.A.D. program's mission and goals.

The mission of our organization, Intermountain Therapy Animals, is to enhance quality of life through the human-animal bond. The mission of Reading Education Assistance Dogs® (R.E.A.D. ®) is a logical extension of that-utilizing the companionship of therapy animals to build and encourage children's love of books and the reading environment, and providing an opportunity for them to practice the full range of communication skills. Research indicates that positive experiences like this will help lay the foundation for a lifetime of learning, and a higher quality life.

How exactly does the R.E.A.D. program work?

In the library setting, it has worked several ways. When we introduced the program in the Salt Lake City main library in November of 1999, it was four weeks of "Dog Day Afternoons." Kids who signed up for appointments, and came to at least three of the four weekly sessions, were rewarded at the end with the privilege of selecting a brand new book to keep, which was then "pawtographed" by their favorite R.E.A.D. dog. This is a good way for a library to start out with a pilot test of the program. Since then, in the Salt Lake main library and five branches, we just have one R.E.A.D. team that spends two hours at each library every Saturday afternoon, and kids can decide spontaneously to read with the dog. It's a fun and popular activity, and would be classified as AAA or an animal-assisted activity. We now think that a special limited-time event, such as four weeks, or a once-a-month event, is the way to go, rather than ongoing indefinitely. It is a fact of human nature that when things stay special, they are appreciated more. When the dogs are an ongoing Saturday afternoon feature at the library, soon other special events start to be scheduled simultaneously, for example.

In the school setting, we ask the teacher or reading specialist to select those children who would most benefit from the program, and teams read with the same children each week, so that a more trusted and secure relationship evolves. This is AAT, or animal-assisted therapy, because specific goals are set for each child, documentation is kept, and progress is recorded. Sometimes this is done right after school; sometimes during the school day, but it involves a one-on-one experience with privacy or semi-privacy so that the child can blossom without the criticism of his/her peers. Each child spends about a half-hour with his dog; a few minutes getting acquainted and comfortable; time reading; then a few minutes at the end for tricks and treats and less formal play. They often sit together on the floor with big pillows, the dog sits or lies nearby, usually with some physical connection between dog and child, and we see what unfolds.

The dog makes a wonderful vehicle for communication. The handler can speak for and about the dog to make many valid points about pronunciation and comprehension. The handler can say, for instance, "Rover has never heard that word before, Jimmy—can you tell him what it means?" The possibilities are endless, and the child feels less embarrassed than when he is put on the spot. Meanwhile there are little games to play-the dog helps turn pages with his paw or nose, the child can give the dog a treat after completing a certain number of pages, etc. We encourage our teams to build on the unique personalities of both dog and handler, so each team develops their own singular "flavor," if you will.

The child is usually petting and stroking the dog while he is reading, which induces relaxation and lowers blood pressure and heart rate. And before you know it, the child forgets how hard he thinks reading is and starts to look forward to it. He comes running in with enthusiasm the next week saying things like: "Oh, Olivia, I have a story today that I know you're just going to love!"

What are the benefits of the R.E.A.D. program?
Some of the documented benefits of therapy with animals include lowering of blood pressure and heart rate, increased relaxation, and a tendency to forget about pain and limitations. A research study almost 30 years ago found that when children get nervous, especially when talking to others, their blood pressure can rise very high, but that if a dog joins the scene, blood pressure will go down very low, whether the child and dog are sitting quietly together or whether the child is reading to the dog. We suspect part of that is because dogs are so trustworthy-people just know they don't have to be self-conscious or worried or embarrassed when they're with a dog.

Remember that even most adults are terrified of public speaking, and most of us have forgotten how daunting it is to have to expound in front of our peers. Often, kids who are learning to read get stressed, not because they aren't capable of reading but because they get nervous and self-conscious, they worry about making mistakes, they worry about looking dumb-and all those worries make it hard to focus. They dread reading in front of their friends, so they often "freeze up" and things just get worse.

When they read with a dog, right away they start to relax, and then they forget about feeling self-conscious or nervous, and pretty soon things start to flow a little better. Before they know it, they are enjoying the experience of reading instead of dreading it, they're even looking forward to the next time. It is simple, and it works beautifully! It also extends beyond the immediate reading experience-many teachers have noted that children who participate in the R.E.A.D. program start to raise their hands and speak out in class when they never could before.

Here are some of the documented benefits of interaction with therapy animals:

Researcher Aaron Katcher notes the following ways that a healthy therapeutic environment is actually created by the presence of an animal. It:

- draws attention outward
- turns off anxiety, anger and depression
- creates safety
- creates intimacy, and
- increases positive expectations of both self and others.

What's more, everyone in the environment experiences these changes—therapists, too!

Other researchers and sources have produced the following exhaustive list: Therapy animals provide comfort; reinforce learning; motivate speech; motivate movement and exercise; stimulate the senses; facilitate counseling; encourage positive social behaviors; foster feelings of safety and acceptance; enhance self-esteem; decrease loneliness; provide the opportunity for touch and for nurturing; provide the opportunity to give instead of receive; inspire people to smile, laugh and have fun; offer unconditional love/acceptance; normalize extremes in a healthy direction; cause people to forget their pain and limitations by focusing outward; provide connections to home and a home-like environment.

Kids learn many things from the animals, in many different ways. One member of our group was a special education teacher whose therapy dog accompanied her to school almost daily. She said she could even use the dog to teach her kids PREPOSITIONS, because they were so fascinated by, and so focused on, the dog that their attention span was much longer, and she could demonstrate things like "about," "beyond," "toward," or whatever, demonstrating with her dog, and the kids would really get it.

As for us with the R.E.A.D. program, all these things are seen. The kids relax into the situation, feel some joy and pleasure in the moment of experience, and begin to look forward to reading instead of focusing on their own inadequacies and dreading the idea.

The wonderful thing about the whole setting is that, just as trouble with reading is usually not a purely intellectual problem, the presence of the dog helps more than reading skills, too. The kids start coming to school more consistently, volunteering to read aloud in class, being late less often, turning in more homework assignments, showing improvements in self-esteem, forming trusting relationships . . . the list just goes on! During the sessions there are unlimited opportunities to discuss things like pet safety, appropriate treatment of pets/animals, personal hygiene, and personal problems. The handlers are often surprised to find themselves in the role of therapist, hearing amazing revelations from these kids, which they then pass on to the proper school representative.

Are they learning about the dogs or are there other messages that come along with it?
Yes, of course. We tend to use books with animal themes so that they are learning in all aspects of the process. They learn about dog behavior, responsible pet care, empathy and feelings, etc. The thing about dogs, and about reading, for that matter, is that NOT being able to read is seldom a purely intellectual problem. In fact, mostly it is a cultural or social or emotional difficulty—we are whole beings, and all the things we need to do and learn are not just isolated skills, but part of a whole context in ourselves. A lot of the kids we have worked with have home problems—domestic violence, or English is their second language, or simple unpredictability and instability, and they bring those problems to school with them, as you know. Dogs always present their whole selves in any situation-no pretense, no holding back, no pretending to be something other than what they are or feel at that moment. That kind of presence is very compelling for people in any therapeutic or learning situation.

So, the kids not only learn to enjoy the reading experience (first of all because the listener is attentive and does not judge or criticize or make fun or tell the child's friends when they make a mistake), then they look forward to it, and then it starts to spill over to other things-they start holding their heads up a little higher, they start coming to school more often, they start completing more homework assignments in other subjects . . . it's really quite remarkable what happens!

How does reading to an animal help raise a child's self-esteem?
There are some obvious ways, such as the fact that lots of focused practice will increase someone's skill and therefore their confidence, and being listened to and treated with respect validates a child and contributes to their self-esteem. There are also some less obvious ways. We soon began to notice that most children consistently turn the book toward the dog so

s/he can see the pictures and understand the story. We learned something important from this, that the kids were getting enormous satisfaction from being the teacher for awhile. Here is someone (the dog) who knows even less about reading than they do, and the opportunity to feel useful and competent, and help someone else understand, really contributes to the child's experience of validation and self-worth. You can almost watch them blossoming in front of your eyes.

One ten-year-old girl we met could hardly read at all—not even as well as an average first-grader. She gave the handler all kinds of reasons why she couldn't and didn't want to read to Meg, the dog. The handler reassured her that Meg wasn't going to be bothered by any of those things, and eventually they sat down to read together. It was a real struggle for this girl, but she became very engrossed in the book and kept at it, with Meg listening beside her. It took her 45 minutes to read just one 32-page picture book with simple words, but when she turned over the to the last page she gasped in happy surprise, "Oh my gosh! I'm finished-I've never read a whole book before, ever in my life!" She got to go home that day with a singular accomplishment. That's the kind of experience that helps to build self-esteem-when someone accomplishes something important, conquers challenges, and feels their skills increasing. The dogs can help support these things in situations where other people, even well-trained, very loving people, somehow can't achieve that important break-through.

How did this program come to be?
Sandi Martin, one of ITA's board members, "put two and two together" by wondering whether therapy animals might be used in the reading setting. A nurse and former ICU manager, she had seen firsthand the benefits that animals brought to patients, and how they helped enhance the desire to heal and work on their therapies. Wouldn't the same benefits accrue with children who were struggling to learn to read? Voila-the idea for Reading Education Assistance Dogs® was born. It's clearly one of those "lightbulb" ideas that seem so brilliant, it's a wonder someone hadn't thought it up long before.

In fact, there is documented evidence that people have read to dogs for a very long time, but Intermountain Therapy Animals was the first to build a structure around this concept and develop it into a true literacy support program with models for schools, libraries and other settings.

Are there any studies in education that support the need for such a program?
The statistics about reading are perennially discouraging. The American Library Association estimates that there are 27 million functionally illiterate adults in the United States. The national "America Reads" program notes that 40% of fourth graders read below their grade level, and that

children who don't master reading by the third grade risk falling further behind. Both Barbara and Laura Bush have been champions of reading. Recently Laura has said, "It's a struggle that affects every American. If our children are not able to read, they are not able to lead." Or learn. Or progress in our society. If you look at Amazon.com, you will see that they list no less than 2,047 nonfiction titles pursuing the critical skill of teaching reading. Despite this outpouring of attention and concern at every level, we don't seem to be making sufficient progress to turn the tide.

What makes the R.E.A.D. program different from the many pet therapy programs?

It may not be different at all, except that occurs in the reading arena instead of a more typical health care institutional setting. In general, we have made a concerted effort to acquaint therapists with the value of AAT and have pushed our interactions way beyond mere visits (though those have therapeutic benefits as well) to serious involvement in the therapeutic regimens of our clients. We push to get the ratio of dog-to-client to one-on-one, because that's where the most powerful changes happen. The same is true for R.E.A.D.—if the children were to sit in a group and take turns reading to the dog that would defeat the whole purpose. Many children fear reading precisely because they are afraid to make mistakes in front of their peers, don't want to be thought stupid, and don't want to be criticized or made fun of for a speech impediment.

What kind of pre/post testing do the R.E.A.D. teams use, especially if the program is considered AAT and documentation is essential?

We find the best way to do testing is to get permission from the school to see the reading scores that the school itself takes periodically. When you have a good collaborative program going, high trust and assurances of confidentiality, school personnel are generally willing to share such results. We feel there is less bias this way-since we don't design the testing process we can't build in biases that favor our outcomes. You can see the progress of the kids who participate in R.E.A.D. right alongside the rest of their classmates' results.

How do you measure the success of the program?

In libraries, they measure it by the kids' enthusiasm and attendance. If they love it, they keep scheduling us again like any successful special event. That's one reason we've decided we prefer not to be a permanent fixture there-it becomes commonplace and therefore less appreciated; with regular, ongoing programs they schedule OTHER special events on top of us sometimes! So now we're cutting back to four-week programs a couple of times per year, or once-a-month sessions.

In schools, we just look at the test scores of the kids who are participating. We figure it's the most credible if we go with the school's own testing instruments. We have a form for that you'll see in the training package, too. Most schools are happy to cooperate with our data-gathering-we just use first names in our records.

What kind of qualities do the R.E.A.D. animals possess?
A good Reading Education Assistance Dog (or cat) is, first of all, a registered, tested and insured therapy animal. This means they have been screened for skills and temperament, health and cleanliness, good manners and attitude. They are animals who people can't resist approaching; they inspire confidence and trust in the people around them. They are calm and reliable, obedient, and impeccably groomed to be attractive and fun to touch and stroke. They enjoy children, and like curling up on the floor with them to hear stories.

What type of animals are involved in the program?
We have dogs of all sizes who participate, from little terriers to giant mastiffs. Temperament is more relevant than size. We also have R.E.A.D. cats, bunnies and guinea pigs for those who prefer the company of alternative creatures. And just recently an African Grey parrot has become a R.E.A.D.er!

Why does it have to be a registered therapy dog and not just a pet? Do you ever use dogs that are from shelters?
We advocate registered therapy animals for many reasons. The testing has shown that each particular animal has the appropriate skills and temperament to do the job; the owner has demonstrated great responsibility and willingness to train and care for their animal; and each animal has liability insurance, which is a great comfort to all concerned-owners, facilities and clients.

Although many of our therapy animals came from shelters to their current homes, we feel that taking animals straight from a shelter to do therapy work is just another source of confusion and stress for those who are already taxed to their limits. It is not fair to shelter animals to be used in that way.

Can my dog and I just do it alone-does there have to be a therapy group in place in my area?
Many people have become the first in their community to register with their animals as a therapy team; there is no reason a R.E.A.D. team could not operate independently, as well. With fewer teams you just see fewer children.

How are your animals trained/tested—by what agency/criteria?
Volunteer therapy teams use many different testing and registering entities. We especially endorse the Delta Society's Pet Partner® program, since it promotes training of both the person and the animal who volunteer

together. After a team goes through the rigors of therapy registration and training, there is an additional workshop and training for R.E.A.D. handlers beyond that. While sitting around comfortably with their owner and a child may come quite naturally to a dog, there are some additional skills that are useful, such as learning to look at a book, being able to focus on the situation amidst many distractions, comfort around the general noises and commotion that can occur in schools, like schoolbells, costumes, puppets, room decorations, etc.

We know the kids benefit from the program—do the dogs benefit as well?

Good question. Most of the dogs truly enjoy spending cozy time with their owner and friends, collecting love, relaxing to the sound of sweet voices, and enjoying some treats. It's important to note that we wouldn't make any dog do this if he weren't having fun, too. It's one of our most serious obligations as the two-legged partner on the team, to make sure our animals are not forced to participate if they don't enjoy the interaction. The animals are not tools or machines, but individuals with their own needs and preferences, and we honor that at every turn.

How much training do your volunteers have?

Our ITA teams start with an eight-hour basic workshop, four hours of more active orientation, an additional three hours of R.E.A.D. training, and then mentoring as they get immersed in the various settings. Some groups have eight- to ten-week training sessions for doing animal-assisted therapy. We rely more on mentoring and on-the-job experience, which the teams seem to remember more effectively and which is more practical for our purposes.

Do the handlers get special reading assistance training? If so, who provides that?

At this time, we do not require that the handler have formal literacy training, but we have an additional three-hour orientation for teams that want to start doing the R.E.A.D. program. We offer a lot of tips and guidance on how to help children learn to read and to enjoy the reading experience. We also offer many additional suggestions developed from our experiences with the animals and how they affect the reading environment.

Often the handler will use projection, communicating through and for the animal, to teach concepts and to help overcome obstacles. This approach is more appealing to the child and more effective because s/he doesn't feel targeted or pressured. For example, if a child reads a word but doesn't know what it means, the handler might say, "Gee, I don't think Rover has ever heard the word 'interactive' before-can you tell him what it means?" If he knows, great; if he doesn't, they can get a dictionary together and learn the new word and explain it to the dog. This is less direct and intimidating than, "Do you know what that word means?" a direct question which a child may shrink from.

A lot of the magic in this program revolves around letting the child focus on the dog. When s/he thinks s/he's helping the dog understand the words and the story, the child gets the empowering feeling of being the helper and teacher-rather than having the whole experience focus on the child's lack of skill. This critical shift in focus makes an incredible difference in the flow of the child's learning processes. It's much more fun to read with a friend who listens attentively, and does not judge, than to read for your teacher, in front of your peers.

How does the presence of the handler not interfere in the child-dog relationship, or inhibit the child reader?
It's been documented in many therapeutic settings that when an animal is present in therapy, people tend to forget about the other humans and their inhibitions disappear. It's why they often are considered powerful bridges for people who are suffering the after-effects of emotional or sexual abuse. They don't trust anyone and won't talk, but when an animal is introduced, they find it trustworthy and suddenly will open up (therapist still present) and talk about lots of things the therapist needs to hear but which they were previously unwilling to share.

Something similar happens in the reading setting. Of course, the handler is ALSO a supportive, positive, uncritical listener. The handler fulfills a crucial role in the process, in encouragement, helping the reader "help the dog understand"—which the kids are eager to do-it takes pressure off them and helps their abilities flow. They also work with comprehension, using the dictionary, etc.

What makes a child eligible for the program?
In the library programs, any interested child (generally K-6) is welcome to read to the animals. Because kids can't really be selected for reading ability, it tends to be a more social and casual way to use the program to help kids have positive experience with books, reading and the library.

In the school programs, children are selected by their teachers and reading specialists as those who would most benefit from this type of intervention-kids who lack confidence, have difficulty with English (especially if they are not native speakers), kids with short attention spans, kids whose reading scores are well below average for their age and grade.

In the classroom setting, we DON'T want kids to think they've been selected or singled out because of their inadequacies-one more thing to make them feel bad. We tend to bring several therapy dogs into the class, give them a presentation about what therapy dogs do in other settings, and then the teacher asks if anyone would enjoy spending time reading with one of these dogs. Usually it's unanimous, and then of course the teachers can select a subgroup of kids who get to do the program and it can be designed to look more like a reward than a remedial program, so they feel special rather than singled-out negatively.

Criteria for selection do not need to be strictly or narrowly defined-it all depends on the facility and the population. One teacher has just one visiting team, and she likes all her first-graders to participate, so they cycle through about five or six children each week and then start all over again, so each child is participating once every five to six weeks. The teacher keeps the handler informed about what each child needs most that week and they work on that together.

And while we initially concentrated on children K-3, we have already been asked to target different groups. In some schools they select older children (grades 4-6) from several classes for an after-school program. The school's reading specialist supervises the group, and the same 10–12 kids come each week to get 20-30 minute sessions with the same dog for a whole semester or whole school year. Three to four teams participate. Their selection criteria include kids who may be suffering from some terrible home situation (split, poverty, domestic violence) and/or kids who are immigrants learning English. In one particular school there were a lot of kids from Bosnia, some of whom have even watched relatives be murdered in front of their eyes, so they're dealing with post-traumatic stress as well.

We have begun a R.E.A.D. program with adolescent boys in a lock-down facility, where we use books with "high interest/low vocabulary." These boys already have damaged egos and don't need to be further patronized by trying to read children's picture books, even though their reading skills are woefully below par. We have been approached by Head Start, and we are planning to work with them to determine how to prepare pre-school kids to look forward to learning to read. There is really no child who couldn't benefit from the R.E.A.D. setting. We even got a letter from one mom who said her daughter is an excellent reader and they go to the library every weekend, but she is really eager to spend time with the dogs because they live in an apartment and can't have pets, so for her, it's the opportunity to hang out with the dogs that just enhances the library experience even more.

Parental approval is always obtained before any child is allowed to participate in the program.
One school told us that a little six-year-old boy walked into the principal's office and stated, "I want to be one of the kids who get to read to the dogs— where do I sign up?" Don't we wish that we had enough teams so everyone who wanted to could be included!

How do you handle various cultural sensitivities?

We try to get relevant information like this from the teacher or staff before ever starting, but sometimes we learn as we go. One little boy always wanted to be around the dogs but he kept his hands clasped behind his back. The handlers, thinking he was perhaps frightened, reassured him that the dogs were friendly and encouraged him to touch them. He replied that is was not permitted, in his religion, to touch animals. The handlers were surprised, but upon asking the teachers found out that, indeed, he belonged to a particular Muslim sect that didn't permit touching animals. The boy continued to be interested in seeing the dogs but very carefully avoided touching them. The parents had given permission for his visual participation, and the handlers respected his boundary.

Do the kids get to choose an animal to read to?

Sometimes. It depends on how many teams are participating in a particular location at a specific time. If only one dog comes, then that's the dog they read with.

Do the kids tend to respond better to a large or small dog?

Everyone has their own preferences; we haven't seen anything that universally favors one over the other. We have dogs ranging from 180 lb. mastiffs to 2 lb. Yorkies, and there is always someone who wants and needs just what each one can offer. Small dogs are nice for curling up in laps, of course, but often small ones are less happy around children, so the preference of the DOG is always of prime importance, as well. With large ones, they themselves can become cushions or reclining rest spots, or they can lay their head in the child's lap. Both provide sensory stimulation. Really, it's ultimately a matter of the right personality, skills and temperament for each situation. Young, active labs are great for rehab patients who need to exercise their arm, or for teenage boys in detention programs who aren't physically disabled but are looking for lots of action and fun. Older, couch-potato types tend to be good for the R.E.A.D. program. The dog who taught special ed kids was a Sheltie, small and agile enough to navigate the classroom, but some Shelties aren't at all comfortable around children . . . See what we mean? There is no standard "right" answer to this one.

Have any of the children had negative reactions to the dogs?

No, not so far! Sometimes children are initially afraid of big dogs, but we can always help them get to know each other and overcome their fears. We never force any interaction, of course.

What about allergies?

Our animals are scrupulously clean and well-groomed before each session, which helps. In addition, they use a wonderful product (Nature's Miracle Dander Remover and Body Deodorizer) which helps to lessen the likelihood of any allergic reaction for several hours. If a child suffers from severe allergies or asthma, the R.E.A.D. program would probably not be appropriate or enjoyable.

How do I select appropriate books to read?

We include a booklist chock-full of appropriate book choices for children of various ages. New books are arriving almost daily, so it's always a great idea to consult with teachers and librarians about the best, most up-to-date choices.

Who chooses the book(s) to read? Does the dog ever bring his favorite stories?

Yes, the dog brings his favorites! Some teams have the kids autograph their dog's favorite book as an ongoing "scrapbook" of memories for themselves. We actually bring a rolling suitcase packed full of books every week, for them to choose from. The teachers and librarians also often have lots of books selected, out on display and available.

But this is another area where pre-discussions with the teacher and/or reading specialist are invaluable. You need to have the right level books for each child-not too hard, not too easy. You need to make sure they don't just read the same one over and over each week so that it gets easier for them in a spurious way. (It helps to take notes on each child-for these reasons, and also because they are so thrilled when you remember things about each one of them from session to session.)

Do you find certain kinds of books are more popular than others? For that matter, do you select the reading material or does the school/library?

Well, we're kind of biased toward books about animals!! And there's certainly no shortage of those. We also try to make sure that the books we use represent animals and our stewardship of them in the most positive way.

We bring along a cache of books in a rolling suitcase, so kids can pick from those if they want. But in school, we also consult with the teacher or reading specialist to make sure we're using books at an appropriate level for each child we work with (not too easy, a bit of a stretch but not so hard they bog down, either). At the library, the librarians are so excited about the program they usually put out a display on the days we're coming. The important thing is to have a good, collaborative relationship going with the staff you work with to help with this sort of thing-at the library it includes having posters and flyers in advance to advertise the program, putting pawprints on the floor the days of the program, etc.

Also, we do have our own NEW books along because, when a child in the school programs completes ten books, we let him select a new book to keep from our stash, and then we have "his" therapy animal pawtograph it for him to keep. There's a study out there that says children who haven't learned to read well often have quite spartan or deprived home situations, and having a new book of their own is a precious commodity that they really appreciate. So we don't use thrift-shop books-we solicit donations of new ones from bookstores, etc. Or get them from grant money.

Does the handler ever read to the child and the dog?
Yes, at the libraries, especially. Some kids are too young to read yet, or too scared, so the handler warms them up by helping. Sometimes a book is a bit too challenging, perhaps, so they take turns reading pages.

We've also had some kindergarten-level kids, so we pack along a few alphabet books (there are lots of them that feature animals!) and even some sponge alphabet letters, if things get that basic. It's kind of a fun variation, actually.

Do many children participate in the R.E.A.D. sessions? How many are allowed at each session?
This varies in every program and setting. The best of all worlds is having just one child at a time reading to each dog.

The whole point of R.E.A.D. is to give each child a private opportunity to practice and enjoy reading, away from his peers. Children who have difficulty reading often fear making mistakes in front of their friends and classmates. They have told us they worry their friends may think they are stupid. With a dog, there is no criticism or judgment, and no laughter if a mistake is made. So it's not so intimidating.

How long and how often do you think is necessary for it to be of real value to the children?
In the libraries, we try to give each child about 15-20 minutes. In the schools, the sessions are usually 20-30 minutes on a weekly basis, including a little warm-up time and maybe a couple of treats and tricks afterwards, if that seems appropriate. Consistency and the building of a trusting relationship are essential to the therapeutic process. When those things are established, the children know they have something to count on and want to rise to the occasion, too, and make sure they don't miss their appointments. Less often makes it hard to establish a pattern and have them remember and look forward to it.

What kind of an environment do you set up for these sessions?
The environment should be comfortable and semi-private—within view for safety's sake but a bit out of sight and earshot of the others. The reading kids sometimes have big floor-sized pillows or beanbag chairs, as well as individual quilts, blankets or pads that the handlers bring in to help define a space for their dog. Positions vary, depending on the three parties involved (child, dog, handler). Sometimes they're down on their tummies,

sometimes the dog has his head in the child's lap, and sometimes the child reclines on the dog.

Do the sessions begin/end with a time to just chat or play with the dog?

Absolutely—it's very important to warm up for the session and assess the child's emotional state, how he is feeling about the dog, etc. Talk about what a therapy dog is; talk about the dog-his breed, where he came from, what he enjoys; talk about the incentives, like earning books; learn a bit about the child. And it's important to have a break at the end, maybe let the child offer a treat to the dog, etc.

That said, we do try to remind our handlers to keep their focus on reading, not on playing tricks or catch or otherwise getting too far off base, which is often very tempting for everyone.

Does it matter if the dog isn't always attentive?

If the dog is restless, moves around a lot and tries to get up frequently, we take a potty break or offer a drink. Occasionally a session must end early if the dog is having a "bad day." Children understand this quite easily.

When a dog falls asleep during a session, sometimes we tell the child that he is just closing his eyes so he can concentrate better on the story. If the dog starts to snore, this doesn't always work! In that situation, one handler told the child that she should feel very proud, because she always read a story to her dog at bedtime to help him go to sleep, and she had managed to be just as effective. The next time it happened, the little girl looked up at the handler with ashy and glowing smile, saying gently, "I read Buster night-night!"

We try to teach the dogs a "focused attention" command (e.g., "Look!") to get them to look straight at the book sometimes. This is effective. But the children get a lot of satisfaction from reclining against the dog, having their arm around him, or just petting and stroking while reading-he doesn't have to be paying attention every moment for the good things to happen.

Is there any reward system in place for progress goals to be met by the students?

Rewards can be any number of things. We have big bone bookmarks, and each week when a child completes a book they put a sticker on their book-mark, or a pawprint stamp, etc. After they've completed ten books, they get to choose a new book from our collection to keep for their very own, and their dog "pawtographs" it for them.

There are studies that show children from deprived backgrounds have very few books, so giving them the opportunity to choose their very own shiny new one, is extremely valuable and influential. We get new books donated, and preferably hardbacks, so they seem really important and substantial (as opposed to used hand-me-downs). It is a big hit.

What are the costs associated with the R.E.A.D. program (like books, uniforms, program costs, advertising)?
The cost to launch a R.E.A.D. program is minimal. First, of course, there is no cost at all to schools and libraries to host programs (see #37). The cost for volunteer participants varies depending on the therapy organization they are licensed with and the policies of their own local group, if they belong to one. There is the cost of the training manual and DVD for each team, and then the cost of a lifetime registration as a R.E.A.D. team. Beyond that, any uniform requirements or R.E.A.D. ID (such as a shirt for the person, bandana for the dog, etc.) vary from group to group. We do advocate new books as rewards for the children (as opposed to used, hand-me-down editions), and those are often donated by various entities. At R.E.A.D. headquarters, we also print a simple educational brochure and offer it to our teams nationwide for a few cents per copy. The success of the program spreads quickly by word of mouth, and usually the demand from schools and libraries far exceeds supply of teams, so there is no need for paid advertising. (Sometimes local groups do place ads to solicit for more volunteers-always the greatest need!)

Is there a cost to schools, libraries or other facilities associated with the program?
The R.E.A.D. program, as all of our animal-assisted therapy programs, is free of charge to all clients and facilities. However, as a nonprofit organization we are always grateful for donations and many facilities do make them. Also, we accept donations of books for the program from various sources.

How do you get funding?
Intermountain Therapy Animals, like all nonprofit organizations, solicits donations from the public to support our work in any way we can—corporations, foundations, and individuals, to carry on our work.

What are your future plans for the R.E.A.D. program?
Simply to keep growing and reaching more children, offering that indispensable one-on-one experience that will lay the foundation for a child's whole life. R.E.A.D. is a deceptively simple model that has shown it really does have efficacy and power to make a positive difference.

At this writing, in less than ten years' time, the program has almost 2,000 registered teams, covering the entire United States, three Canadian provinces, Europe and beyond. R.E.A.D. has also been selected by Public Television (PBS) as a national educational outreach partner in conjunction with the September 2008 debut of their new series based on the Martha Speaks series of books. We never imagined this when we set forth in November of 1999, but we certainly know now that this is a reasonable and worthy accomplishment and recognition, considering the passionate commitment of all these volunteer teams and the joy we have watched light up the lives of children everywhere.

DOCUMENT 6: FAQ INDEX-PET SUITABILITY FOR THERAPY SERVICE

> Intermountain Therapy Animals. "What Makes an Animal (and Handler)
> Suitable to be a Therapy Animal Team." http://www.therapyanimals.org/
> Pet-Suitability.html (accessed July 1, 2010). Copyright © 1996–2009 by
> Intermountain Therapy Animals. All rights reserved. Reprinted by permission of Intermountain Therapy Animals.

What Makes an Animal (and Handler) Suitable to be a Therapy Animal Team?

Intermountain Therapy Animals looks for very specific qualities in the companion animals it registers as therapy animals. Pet owners who are considering signing up to be animal-assisted therapy handlers should keep the following in mind:

What Kinds of Animals Will Qualify?

Besides dogs and cats, there are a great many other species that make wonderful visiting animals and can form strong human-animal bonds. To name just a few: birds, rabbits, goats, domestic rats, hamsters, guinea pigs, ducks and chickens, goats, miniature pigs, llamas, cows and horses.

At this time, Intermountain Therapy Animals does not work with large animals like llamas, cows and horses. (But if this is your interest, stay tuned, because there may be another group organizing locally quite soon that will specialize in large animals in a farm-like setting.) Also, animals such as snakes, ferrets, lizards and wild or exotic animals are not registered. This is because wild or exotic animals are not legally acceptable as pets in many states, and without more research documenting their predictability over time, we cannot accurately evaluate their behavior and reaction to stress.

What Makes an Animal Appropriate?

Animals should have at least a basic level of training so that they are reliable and under control even in crowded situations and when there are loud noises. Therapy animals should convey the image that they are well-behaved and have good manners. Because we love our animals, it is important that animals who participate in AAA/AAT have an interest in people and enjoy visiting. Look at the following checklist about what makes an animal appropriate for AAA/AAT.

- Animal demonstrates behavior that is reliable, controllable, predictable, and inspires confidence in the person s/he is interacting with
- Animal actively solicits interactions with people and is accepting and forgiving of differences in people's reactions and behavior
- Animal demonstrates relaxed body posture, moments of sustained eye contact (dependent upon species and breed), and relaxed facial expressions
- Animal is more people-oriented than animal-oriented
- Animal likes being petted, touched and hugged
- Animal is able to remain calm with people doing such things as speaking loudly, clumsy movements and clapping
- When approached from the rear, the animal may show curiosity, but does not startle, growl, jump up, bark, eliminate, act shy or resentful
- The animal can walk on various surfaces reasonably comfortably, including carpet, concrete or asphalt, tile, linoleum, rubber matting and wooden floors
- Animal can be held by another person than its owner for several minutes, continuing to demonstrate good manners with no vocalizing or extreme nervousness
- Animal is outgoing, friendly and confident in new settings

What Kinds of Animals Definitely Will NOT Qualify?

- Any pet that is aggressive to people or other animals would not pass the tests. Growling, snapping, lunging, extended barking, raising of hackles, or bearing of teeth will disqualify a dog. Sometimes we meet owners who tell us, when their dog starts to growl, that "he's just talking," or "that's just his way to say hello." Even if that's true, it doesn't work to have an animal in school and hospital settings, with people who are sick and perhaps frightened or even tentative about meeting a dog, to have to recoil in fear.
- If your pet is in poor health it would not be safe for it or the people s/he meets to be exposed. We visit in situations that are very fragile medically, and therapy animals must be picture-perfect in both health and grooming.
- If your animal is unpredictable (sweet one moment, aggressive the next) or doesn't like being around people (shy, backs away, gets nervous, quivers, etc.) it would not be suitable.
- We do not accept any dogs who are wolf hybrids, even though many are wonderful companions, again because they can be unpredictable.
- It is very important for your pet to live like a member of your family. Most dogs who live most of their lives outdoors, especially if they sleep outside and/or are kept chained most of the time, do not

make good therapy animals. Dogs who are well behaved, well socialized members of their pack are most successful as therapy dogs.

What, Specifically, Will You and Your Animal Have to Do During the Test?

Essentials: You must pass all these skill-test items to qualify:

- Your dog must be accepting of a friendly stranger and be willing to sit politely for petting. Must also be clean, healthy and well-groomed.
- Your dog must be willing to go "out for a walk" with you on a loose lead—no pulling or dragging! Then you must both walk through a crowd, also on a loose leash, and be subjected to several visual and noise distractions without your dog panicking, becoming aggressive or too submissive.
- Basic obedience: your dog will have to do a sit, a down, a stay-in-place, and a come-when-called. It must be able to meet a neutral dog without overreacting.

Aptitudes: You may score "not ready" on no more than three of these and still pass:

- Generally, these items relate to people, equipment and situations that you and your animal may encounter while doing therapy visits. Your dog must not object to a thorough, all-over handling by a stranger (fingers in mouth, on tail, feet, etc.), a restraining hug, a staggering, gesturing individual, angry yelling going on, crowded petting, wheelchairs, walkers, etc. Your dog must also be willing to be held by a stranger for two minutes while you disappear. This test grades for overall sociability and observes carefully how must your dog is enjoying this sort of activity. *We do not want to try to do good in the world if it means making our animal companions miserable.*

These test items are primarily for dogs. If you have some other animal, there will be some variation in the procedures to accommodate species differences.

DOCUMENT 7: OBEDIENCE AND YOUR THERAPY ANIMAL BY CONNIE SHARKEY AND KATHY KLOTZ

Intermountain Therapy Animals. "Basic Obedience and Your Therapy Animal." http://www.therapyanimals.org/documents/Obedience%20and%20Your%20Therapy%20Animal%202.2010.pdf (accessed July 1, 2010).

People often say to us, "I have a new puppy (or a new adoptee) and I want it to be a therapy dog. What do I have to do?"

There is no guarantee that your dog will want to be a therapy dog—that is, have the innate desire to engage with people outside his own pack, enjoy the activities and cope with the potential stresses associated with patient/ clients in various settings. We urge you to consider your dog's needs and preferences in this regard. Still, there are many things you can do to maximize the chances that your dog will have excellent potential as a visiting companion.

First Things First: How Important Is Training?

Long before you consider making an investment in time and education for therapy visits, raise your pup to be a well-behaved companion in all of your family and household activities. Ask yourself some questions about the relationship you and your dog will have in "regular" life: What do you want your dog's role to be? How active or sedentary is your lifestyle? Where will you want your dog to accompany you—around town doing errands in the car? To your workplace? On long walks or camping and hiking adventures? What will you want your dog to do in each and every setting?

As a pack animal, your dog is hard-wired to want to know where s/he fits in, what you expect and what his/her job is going to be. Dogs are extremely flexible and adaptable—no other species on our planet has proven so malleable as the dog, which now has more than 400 distinct breeds. So, no matter what your ultimate goals, the first essential is to TRAIN. Training is much more than specific commands—it includes clear and consistent communication about your boundaries, rules, preferences and expectations. In other words, building your relationship and teaching appropriate skills for the life you and your dog will lead together. *Training is simply the greatest gift you can give your dog*, so that you can be proud to include her in your life, which is where she wants to be. She will love that far more than fashion accessories, a fluffy dog bed or a giant yard.

The Basics for Every Dog

You and your dog will go a long way, either in everyday life or in therapy volunteering, with the basics: sit, down, stay, come, and walking on a loose lead. And there are multiple philosophies out there about how to achieve these skills. If you and your dog have never taken an obedience class together, consider doing it now. It is never too late. Ideally, start with a puppy kindergarten class. Read some books and watch trainers on TV. There are many excellent books and training shows available.

Skills YOU Need to Train Effectively

Guess what? YOU need to have some skills in order to train your dog—skills that make it easy for your dog to understand what you want.

Be the Leader

This is the basis for everything else. All dogs want to know who's in charge, and they respond well to demonstrated leadership. Many professional trainers say that lack of leadership accounts for most problems people have with their dogs. When dogs do not see a strong leader, they assume they must try to step up and take that role! Being the leader doesn't mean being a yelling dictator—it means being confident, calm, clear and authoritative. One easy way to do this: do not ask, beg or cajole your dog for what you want—tell him. Not only with your voice, but also with your attitude and body posture.

Be Interesting

Be more interesting and exciting to your dog than anything else in the immediate environment. Be animated, use different tones of voice and pacing, use your dog's favorite motivators, like food or toys (see "Right Equipment," below), so that she will want to focus on you and what you're asking.

A Bunch of C Words: Communication, Consistency, Clarity

How do you communicate with your animal so that it understands what you are attempting to teach it? Be crisp and clear, and don't keep repeating yourself. When you say the command again, again, and again, you are only conveying that you really don't expect the behavior until you have asked many times, and you will both end up frustrated.

Be consistent with your commands and body language. If you ask for a sit by saying the word "sit" and showing the dog what "sit" means with food, and then rewarding the dog when its rear hits the ground, you have made progress toward teaching your dog to sit. However, if you use several different words, or say the same word several times, or fail to let your dog know when it has achieved your desire, then once again you wind up frustrated and your dog is unhappy because it knows it hasn't pleased you, but it's not sure why.

Right Equipment

Appropriate equipment can make all the difference in training an animal. Start with a collar and a leash. Harnesses may be useful or desirable after your dog knows what you want, but they make it much harder to communicate to your dog what you are attempting to teach it. In therapy work you cannot use choke chains, any collar made of metal, or prong/pinch collars, so don't become dependent on those if therapy visiting is your goal. Use a good nylon or leather buckle collar or a head collar for extra control, and a 5-6' leash. Use a different collar for training than the one used for going for walks or playing. Dogs pick up on this really fast and know when it's time for work. You'll also need a motivator—anything that causes your dog to understand that you are happy with what he has done. Use food (small bits of whatever your dog most loves) or a favorite toy. The motivator is used to entice your dog into the desired position and then to reward it for achieving that position.

Timing

When I tell my dog to sit, I show my dog, by making it lift its head, that I want its bottom to hit the ground. Then I immediately give it praise just as its bottom hits the ground. In this way, I have timed my positive reinforcement so that it has meaning to my dog, and he knows he has done what I wanted.

Giving Corrections

It is also important to know how and when to use correction. A correction is not punishment or pain, it is the level of compulsion necessary to get your dog's attention. The amount of compulsion needed may increase as the level of distraction increases. But as with positive reinforcement, a correction must be given instantly, not two or five minutes later. Use a consistent word, sound or hand signal. "No" is most obvious but not necessarily most effective. Try a cheerful "uh-uh" or "oops."

Take Baby Steps and Build Slowly

For each new skill you begin to train, remember baby steps. Letting your dog know what behavior you want is your biggest challenge. Get your dog to do the desired behavior, then "name it and claim it." Stay focused, and if you or your partner is having a bad day, stop and try again later. During the day, you can always throw in random requests for a come, sit, down, etc. as you go about your daily activities.

Keep Training Sessions Short and Frequent

One of our favorite bits of training advice is to train three or four times a day, but only 5-10 minutes each session. That way it's fun for both of you—your dog never gets tired or bored, and you really can't claim that you have no time to train your dog!

Train in Many Different Environments

If you only request a sit in the kitchen, your dog won't necessarily respond out in the backyard. Get them accustomed to the sights, sounds, smells, surfaces and distractions of different environments, as well as to all kinds and sizes of people.

Important Skills to Teach Your Dog for Therapy Visiting

Your success in therapy volunteering will pivot on your relationship with your dog and your skills as a team. Once you master the methods, you will be amazed how easily your dog can learn, and how much fun he will have learning new skills and pleasing you.

The ideal therapy dog is calm, friendly, easily controllable, and predictable, and has a demeanor that inspires confidence in others. To visit clients effectively and successfully, you will need to provide a companion who can walk with you on a loose lead and respond to your requests. You will need to have a trusting relationship and be highly attuned to one another. When your dog trusts you and responds to your requests, you can both be confident and comfortable in various visit environments.

In therapy work, mastering the basic commands is essential for several reasons, no matter the size or personality of your dog, or the length of his legs. First, they will show that your dog can be calm, responsive and controllable, in all situations; next, they will be a good indicator of the relationship and bond between the two of you; and, not least, your clients will be delighted when they can ask your dog to do any of those things and get a positive response.

Unlike formal competition obedience, we suggest softer tones and smaller, more subtle signals, and— very importantly—you may constantly offer your dog guidance, reassurance and support.

Additional Skills Useful in Therapy Settings

Teach your dog to *wave* or offer a *high-five*. Your clients will love it and ask for it every time!

Another useful skill is for your dog to *sit politely by your side* until you let him know he may move forward to meet a new person. This will give you time to make sure a visit is welcome from the person you are approaching. Or, in the case of a child, you have time to ask a parent if a visit will be appreciated.

A *leave it* (use whatever words you prefer) is extremely valuable because you don't want your dog floor surfing for leftover food, or even pills, that are often present in care facilities.

Beyond these, almost anything your dog knows how to do can be incorporated into a visiting setting. For example, one little dog we know loves to dance on his hind legs. He likes to accompany patients with walkers. When normally they may struggle to accomplish a goal of six feet or ten feet, if Tippy accompanies them, they enjoy watching his dancing so much that they may walk 12 feet or 20 feet without even noticing, because they don't want the fun to end.

Reap the Rewards

If your dog loves to interact with humans beyond his own pack, and has learned the basic commands, volunteering as a visiting therapy team may be just the ticket for you both. When you get out your visit bag and uniform and your dog starts getting excited to go, you will know that your dog is eagerly anticipating his "job" and you can both look forward to satisfying and rewarding adventures in therapy work.

DOCUMENT 8: CANINE COMPANIONS FOR INDEPENDENCE–HOW SHOULD PEOPLE BEHAVE AROUND AN ASSISTANCE DOG?

Canine Companions for Independence. "How Should People Behave Around an Assistance Dog?" http://www.cci.org/site/c.cdKGIRNqEmG/ b.4011011/k.F407/Etiquette.htm (accessed July 1, 2010). © 2008 by Canine Companions for Independence, Inc. All rights reserved. Reprinted by permission of Canine Companions for Independence.

How should people Behave Around an Assistance dog?

The Americans with Disabilities Act guarantees people with disabilities the right to be accompanied by a service animal in all areas open to the general public. Service animal means any assistance dog or other animal individually trained to do work or perform tasks for the benefit of an individual with a disability. Here are some tips to follow when meeting or approaching a working assistance dog and his or her partner:

- *Don't be afraid of the dog.* Assistance dogs from organizations like Canine Companions for Independence and other members of Assistance Dogs International are carefully tested and selected for appropriate temperament. They have been professionally trained to have excellent manners.
- *Don't touch the dog without asking permission first!* This is a distraction and may prevent the dog from tending to the human partner.
- *Never feed the dog.* It may be on a special diet. CCI dogs are generally on a feeding schedule as well. Food is the ultimate distraction to the working dog and can jeopardize the working assistance dog team.

- *Speak to the person, not the assistance dog!* Most handlers do not mind talking about assistance dogs and their dog specifically if they have the time.
- *Do not whistle or make sounds to the dog* as this again may provide a dangerous distraction.
- *Never make assumptions about the individual's intelligence, feelings or capabilities.*
- *Be aware of potential architectural barriers to the individual.* Be respectful of the assistance dog team. They are a working pair going about their daily lives.

Business owners: Some customers and employees may be anxious or nervous about an assistance dog in your establishment. Reassure them that the dog is thoroughly trained and has a legal right to be there under the ADA. People with assistance dogs deserve the same respect as any other customer.

Document 9: Code of Ethics the Israeli Association of Animal-Assisted Psychotherapy

This document was written by the Committee for the Creation of a Professional Code of Ethics for Animal-Assisted Psychotherapy in preparation for the establishment of the IAAAP. The committee was chaired by Tamar Axelrod and included Tamar Axelrad-Levy, Tamar Chazut, Sari Bar-On, Shirli Shani, Michal Tibika-Nadjar, and Hanita Yehoshua (http:// www.cci.org/site/c.cdKGIRNqEmG/b.4011011/k.F407/Etiquette.htm accessed July 1, 2010). © by The Israeli Association of Animal-Assisted Psychotherapy. All rights reserved. Reprinted by permission of the Israeli Association of Animal-Assisted Psychotherapy.

Training and Professional Responsibility

1. One will be considered an Animal-Assisted Psychotherapist if one has fulfilled the requirements of professional academic and field training according to the requirements determined by the Israeli Association of Animal-Assisted Psychotherapy, and in the future according to requirements determined through the recognition of a governmental body.
2. The AAP therapist is expected to be aware of his/her responsibilities and obligations.
3. The AAP therapist is expected to maintain a high professional level and to keep updated with professional developments and new ideas–both in the areas of mental health and of animals.
4. The AAP therapist is expected to act fairly and respectfully towards clients and also towards other professionals, to cooperate with them for the good of the client, to not libel or discriminate on the basis of age, sex, race or religion.

5. The AAP therapist is expected to be acquainted with the various animals with which (s)he works (the animal's life style, needs, abilities and limitations) in the therapy context, and to be considerate of the animal's needs, and to be aware that (s)he is responsible for the animal's welfare.

6. The AAP therapist is expected to be aware of the unique characteristics of this type of therapy:

   a. The animal's vitality is a factor that initiates events that create and influence the therapy dynamics.

   b. The live animal's presence in the session creates various therapeutic connections with various characteristics

   therapist ↔ client
   therapist ↔ animal
   client ↔ animal
   animal ↔ animal
   therapist ↔ client ↔ animal

   c. The animal may intensify experiences, emotions, senses.

   d. The animal may invite touch and make it legitimate.

   e. The animal may in many instances facilitate, invite, catalyze creation of emotional connection.

   f. The animal may arouse preoccupation with primary needs: nourishment, love, nurturing, containing, and holding.

   g. The animal may serve as an aid in the development of empathy and concern for others.

   h. The animal may serve as an aid in distinguishing between self and others, and the establishing of a self-identity.

   i. Animals may facilitate regressive and playful expression.

   j. Animals may represent for the client his/her drive-related characteristics (aggression, sexuality).

   k. Animals may serve as an object for projection.

   l. Animals may facilitate experiences of control, capability, success and achievement.

   m. Animals may facilitate reparative experiences that compensate for negative experiences and deprivations from the past.

   n. Animals may serve as a factor in the mobilization of ego strength (selfcontrol, self-restraint, self-regulation, functioning).

7. The AAP therapist must obey the Code of Ethics of the professional association and the regulations of the Ethics Committee.

8. The AAP therapist must obey the national laws related to work in the field of mental health, welfare and education as well as in the field of animal welfare law and its derivations.

9. The AAP therapist must maintain professional contact, for the purpose of supervision, consultation and evaluation, with professionals in the areas of mental health, welfare, education, veterinary science, and animal behavior, according to the framework and population with which one works.

10. The AAP therapist must evaluate, give therapy and supervises only in the area of his/her expertise and according to his/her training and experience in the area of AAT.
11. The AAP therapist must make known to the client (or to the client's guardian) at the time of acquaintance his/her training, skills, professional rank, expertise and experience.
12. The AAP therapist must properly document the therapy process, and be ready to write a professional report on the therapy when required. The report must be adapted in order to be suited to the particular destination of the report (family, educational institution, other therapy professionals). In special cases (such as in the abuse of animals or people or in other dangerous situations), the reporting will be done with in consultation with other professionals appropriate to the situation, and special discretion will be used in order to safeguard the secrecy of the report.
13. Private work:
    a. It is forbidden for the AAP therapist employed by a public institution to work privately within said institution and/or with the same clients, unless one has received special permission to do so from the institution.
    b. The AAP therapist must wait one year between doing therapy with a client within said institution and continuing therapy with that same client privately, unless it is done as part of a special agreement that condones the immediate continuation of the therapy.
14. The AAP therapist must be aware of situations which require the cessation of therapy or the transferring of the client to different psychotherapist in the case of personal limitations.
15. The AAP therapist must know how to terminate the therapy relationship at the appropriate time in a fitting manner and to aid in the transfer of the client to another psychotherapist if needed.
16. The AAP therapist is subject to the authorization and the limitations of the Israeli Association of Animal-Assisted Psychotherapy according to his/her therapy training, specialization and experience.
17. The AAP therapist is obligated to work under supervision and guidance according to the requirements of the Israeli Association of Animal-Assisted Psychotherapy and according to the accepted regulations of the therapist's place of employment.
18. The AAP therapist that has had the proper training and is interested in giving supervision is obligated to fulfill the conditions, including receiving supervision on one's work as supervisor, according to the regulations of the Israeli Association of Animal-Assisted Psychotherapy.
19. Supervisor and educator:
    a. A supervisor or educator must abstain from taking advantage of his/her influential status over his/her intern or supervisee.
    b. A supervisor must abstain from a therapeutic connection with his/her intern or supervisee, unless there is a contract or agreement the otherwise on the part of both sides.

    c. An educator is forbidden to form a therapeutic connection with his/her student or intern.

    d. A supervisor or educator must abstain from creating a therapeutic connection with a client of his/her intern or supervisee without the agreement of all concerned.

    e. A supervisor or educator must be aware of the possible difficulties of creating a therapeutic connection with a client of a past intern or supervisee.

20. The AAP therapist that is also a supervisor or educator is obligated to nurture the professional development of his/her interns and supervisees over time. (S)he must stand as a personal example in the areas of ethics, scholarliness, professional level, and interpersonal attitude in a way that shows respect towards the profession as well as towards his/her clients.

21. The AAP therapist must be sure to, to the best of his/her ability, explain the essence of his/her profession to the public and to professional organizations in Israel and abroad, as well as to do one's best to promote and advance the profession and the Israeli Association of Animal-Assisted Psychotherapy.

Responsibility towards Clients

22. The AAP therapist must act in the best interest of the client and use therapy interventions that are appropriate for the client's needs. The therapist must match the framework of therapy, as well as the therapy contract, to the client, through mutual understanding between the therapist and the client.

23. The AAP therapist must define the therapy contract with the client during the intake with the client: therapy conditions, mutual responsibility, meeting schedule, information concerning therapeutic work with animals, information concerning immunity and legal obligation to report abuse to the proper authorities.

24. The AAP therapist must take into account the medical, psychiatric, neurological and/or psychological state of the client during the therapy process.

25. The AAP therapist must abstain from taking advantage of his/her influential status over the client.

26. It is forbidden for the AAP therapist to do therapy with someone with whom (s)he had family/friendship/economic ties. It is forbidden for the AAP therapist to do therapy with a student for at least two years after the completion of the student's course of studies.

27. The AAP therapist must take care of the emotional welfare of the client while in the presence of animals:

    a. It is forbidden to bring together the animal with the client against the client's will, other than in special cases in which the therapy demands such according to the therapy contract and there is an agreement with the client ahead of time.

    b. It is forbidden to obligate the client against his/her will to touch the animal, other than in special cases in which the therapy demands such according to the therapy contract and there is an agreement with the client ahead of time.

c. Enough space should be provided within the therapy setting to allow for both the client and animal enough space to be comfortable while allowing the client the option of keeping the distance (s)he desires from the animal.

d. Throughout the meeting between the client and the animal, the AAP therapist must be aware of every change or process relating to the condition of the client in relation to the animal.

28. The AAP therapist must worry about the physical welfare of the client while in the presence of animals:

a. Before the first meeting with the client in the presence of the animals:

1. It must be verified that the client does not have any allergies or sensitivities to any animals, or to any specific animals, or to their secretions or to their food.

2. It is advisable to draft a form to assess the medical condition of the client, to be filled in and signed together with the doctor. In the case that there are special risks, one must try to obtain written medical permission for the therapy.

3. In the case of special sensitivities/allergies/immunological issues/cancer/Aids or any other condition in which the client is physically sensitive or vulnerable (including sensitivities to medicine), one must seek a doctor's advice and obtain medical permission according to the risk involved.

4. In the case that it is not possible to obtain written medical permission, one must inform the client (or guardian) of the risks, and have him/her sign a form giving informed consent for the therapy, or alternatively to consider refusing to do therapy.

5. When the need arises (e.g. riding therapy, dolphin therapy), one much check the client's general medical condition and physical fitness specifically in terms of the field of therapy, and to obtain medical permission relevant to the client's condition and to the risks involved.

b. Throughout the therapy:

1. One must stay aware of and check out any signs of allergies or sensitivities to any animals, or to their secretions or to their food.

2. One must not allow the client to do anything that might constitute for him/her possible danger or harm by the animal or by any accompanying accessories, without warning ahead of time of expected dangers (e.g. poking fingers between the bars of the animal's cage, lifting cages).

3. One must not expose the client to an animal with a zoonotic disease.
4. One must not allow the client to touch or get close to an aggressive animal or one that is not used to contact with humans.
5. One must not expose the client to an animal with whom (s) he is unacquainted, to avoid injury (physically or emotionally) towards the client, therapist, animal, group, or the surroundings.
6. In the case that the client is injured by the animal, one must act according to the regulations of the Health Ministry. In addition, on must act according to the following:
   a. give the appropriate basic first aid
   b. report to the person responsible for the client (when relevant) – parent, teacher, director of institution, etc.)
   c. refer the client to a doctor to check for the need for tetanus shot and/or other treatment
   d. isolate of the animal as ruled by law
   e. in each case of a client's injury caused by an animal, one must file a report and inform the authorities according to law relevant to the type of injury.
   f. It is forbidden to allow the client to injure an animal. In the case that the client injures or kills an animal, one must act on two levels: according to the regulations of the Health Ministry, and concerning the client according to the situation that occurred.
29. The AAP therapist must make sure that the therapeutic area, the resources and the methods are appropriate for the client and his/her specific needs:
    a. One must avoid exposing the client to dangers in the environment (therapy room, zoo, gardens, open area, etc.) without proper guidance and supervision.
    b. The therapist must match the environment of the therapy to the needs and limitations (physical, emotional, cognitive) of the client.
    c. The therapist must be especially aware of any possible changes throughout the therapy. The therapist must react immediately and appropriately to any change.
30. The therapist must show professional judgment in choosing the appropriate animal for the client:
    a. according to the therapy goals;
    b. according to the client's age, developmental stage, motor capabilities, and emotional and cognitive sensitivities;
    c. according to the therapy environment.

Multicultural Aspects

31. The AAP therapist must readily accept the complexity and the diversity of his/her clients and of their opinions towards assisting them in therapy.
32. The AAP therapist will not force his/her beliefs about the animals, or his/her manner of working with the animals, onto the client.
33. The AAP therapist should make an effort to acquaint him/herself, as much as possible, with a variety of cultures, traditions, religions, belief systems, values and ecological and geographical environments in order to be able to help a wide variety of clients, through an understanding of their motivations and behaviors during therapy.
34. The AAP therapist must be aware of his/her own beliefs, opinions and prejudices, as well as of the clients' beliefs, opinions and prejudices, before (s)he commences therapy. In addition, one must be aware of their implications on the therapy process and on the dynamics between the therapist and his/her clients and the animals present in therapy.
35. The AAP therapist must be acquainted with the cultural characteristics and symbolism associated with the animals as a therapy tool, and as a source for communication that is not language-dependent.

Closeness, Sexuality, Touch and Intimacy

36. The framework of AAP creates closeness and intimacy – physical and emotional –between the therapist and the client, between the client and him/herself, between the client and the animals, and among the animals. Likewise, activity with the animals (who are, by their very existence, alive and driven by their instincts) is related to a great extent to basic drives and physical closeness. Since this subject is especially sensitive in AAP, the therapist is required to pay attention to this in supervision.
37. The therapist must know how to discern between expressions of sexuality and a close relationship, touch (physical or emotional) and intimacy within the therapy triangle (therapist-client-animal), which are meaningful for the client's personal development, for the therapy process and for the therapy connection. In addition, the therapist must discern between positive close relationships, touch and intimacy on the one hand, and erotic relations and the abuse of close relationships on the other hand, which constitute a grave ethical violation.
38. In the case that unnecessary touch occurred within therapy, the therapist must be sure to bring the subject to supervision and work it through, and later do the same with the client.
39. Coming face-to-face in therapy with animals, which are intrinsically alive and driven by their instincts, brings up in a very tangible way various content (parenthood, birth, nursing, sexuality, mating, violence, etc.) that are likely to bring up difficulties for certain clients. The therapist must be aware of this and make sure that no damage is caused to the client.

40. In reference to touch:

    a. The presence of an animal in therapy invites closeness and awakens feeling of primary needs in the client. One of them is the need for touch.

        1. Closeness by definition is proximity, being located next to someone or something.

        2. Touch by definition is physical contact, the bringing close of a hand or other body part to someone or something.

    b. The therapist must be aware of and differentiate between situations in which

        1. the good of the client demands closeness and contact, while exercising caution and keeping limits,

        2. situations in which closeness and touch are not needed.

    c. In the field of Animal-Assisted Psychotherapy there exist various situations that demand minimal contact between the therapist and the client, between the therapist and the animals, between the client and the animals, between clients, and between the various animals. The therapist must be aware of such and must inform the client (and when needed, those responsible for the client) ahead of time and define this in the therapy contract. The therapist must pass judgment in the following situations:

- the handing of the animal over from therapist to client and between the clients;
- the therapist instilling n the client various skills needed in working with animals, such as: correcting holding, patting, grooming, caring for a wounded animal, etc. (by the therapist or by clients);
- the therapist helping clients who have difficulty touching animals (due to motor disabilities, discomfort, etc.);
- the therapist physically separating the animal from the client in times of distress or danger of either one (in situations of sudden fear or physical harm);
- the therapist physically calming the client due to an emotionally distressing incident with the animal (as in the case of death, sickness, bites, scratches, etc.);
- the therapist giving first aid to the client due to being wounded by an animal;
- the therapist preventing the fall of an animal while the animal is resting on the client;
- the therapist preventing the client from stumbling or falling while in the zoo or trying to get to an animal (the area of the zoo contains cages of various sizes, stairs, railings, barriers, fences, etc.);

- touch is likely between those present in the zoo when the client is interested in getting close to a cage or a certain animal in an especially crowded area;
- a therapeutic intervention involving touch is likely for therapy or rehabilitation purposes, according to the therapist's ethical judgment.
  - d. Within the framework of AAP, the therapist must allow the client to chose the type of touch and proximity to the animal with whom (s)he feels comfortable.
  - e. The therapist must allow enough room in the therapy setting for the client and animals to move around, in such a way that neither the client nor the animal will feel threatened.
  - f. The therapist must allow the client to decided to which animals (s)he wants to be exposed.
  - g. The therapist must avoid forcing the client to touch an animal.
  - h. The therapist must be aware of and avoid touch that may hurt the client or the animal.
  - i. The therapist must avoid allowing touch with or proximity to an animal that is potentially harmful or that is not used to humans.
  - j. The therapist must avoid exposing the client to animals with which the therapist is not acquainted, so as to prevent injury (physical or emotional) to the client, the therapist, the animal or the surroundings.
41. In reference to sexuality between the therapist and the client:
  - a. The therapist is forbidden to be involved in a sexual relationship with a client and/or supervisee.
  - b. The therapist is forbidden to be involved in erotic activity with a client and/or supervisee.
  - c. The therapist is forbidden to undress in the presence of a client and/or supervisee.
  - d. The therapist is forbidden to allow the client to undress for the purpose of self-exposure.
  - e. The therapist is forbidden to have a sexual relationship with a former client after the conclusion of therapy.
  - f. The therapist should take care to avoid the legitimizing of inappropriate closeness as a result of misinterpretation due to the need for closeness by the therapist, by the client, or by both.
42. In reference to sexual content that arises in therapy:
  - a. The therapist must be aware of the power of animals and of the fact that they bring up in a very concrete way sexual content that is likely to be problematic for certain client.
  - b. The therapist must apply judgment, in each case, according to the condition of the client, as to whether to allow the client's presence during events and experiences of a sexual nature.

43. In reference to intimacy:
   a. Intimacy by definition is closeness, family, friendship, camaraderie
   b. The therapist must be aware that the presence of animals may fundamentally influence the development of intimacy and beware of its consequences.
   c. The therapist must be aware of and differentiate between:

      1. the strength of positive motivation related to intimacy that is due to the three-way therapy relationship and interactions of therapist/client/animal;
      2. the misuse of intimacy that may cause confusion and blurring of limits.

DOCUMENT 10: BENEFICIAL EFFECTS OF PET RELATIONSHIPS: RESULTS OF A PILOT STUDY IN ITALY

Capone F., Bompadre G., Cinotti S., Alleva E., Cirulli F. "Beneficial Effects of Pet Relationships: Results of a Pilot Study in Italy" in Vitale A., Laviola G., Manciocco A., Adriani W. (Ed.). Course. Human and non-human animals interaction: contextual, normative and applicative aspects. Istituto Superiore di Sanita. December 18–19, 2006. Roma: Istituto Superiore di Sanita; 2007. (Rapporti ISTISAN 07/40). p. 74–84. http://www.iss.it/binary/publ/cont/07-40.1197018941.pdf. Reprinted with permission.

Some General Concepts on Human-Animal Relationships

At the end of the last Ice Age, the transition from hunting-gathering to farming favoured the process of animal domestication. The first species to make the transition from a wild to a domestic state was the wolf (*Canis lupus*) and its domestication was based on a mutually beneficial relationship with man. Until recently, archaeological findings were the only evidence to pinpoint the beginning of man's symbiotic relationship with dogs, the commonly accepted date of dog's domestication being placed at 14,000 to 10,000 years ago.

However, some anthropologists suggest that the human-dog relationship could be almost as old as modern man himself.[1] In return for companionship and food, the early ancestor of the dog assisted man in tracking, hunting, guarding and a variety of other purposes. Eventually man began to selectively breed these animals for specific traits. Physical characteristics changed and individual breeds began to take shape. As man wandered across Asia and Europe, he took his dogs with him, using them for additional tasks and further breeding them for selected qualities that would better enable them to perform specific duties.

One of the most important aspects of the domestication of canids has to do with the selection of social-communicative skills.[2] As an example, dogs are more skilful than great apes at a number of tasks in which they must read human communicative signals. Furthermore, wolves raised by humans do not show the same skills as domestic dogs, including puppies that have had little human contact. These findings suggest that during the process of domestication, dogs have been selected for a set of social-cognitive abilities that enable them to communicate with humans in unique ways.[3] Thus, dogs able to use social cues to predict the behaviour of humans more flexibly than could their last common wolf ancestor have been at a selective advantage.

Despite the efforts of generations of ethnologists and psychobiologists, until recently animals have not being recognized to possess a "mind". Historically, cognitive ethnologists gained scientific acceptance between the end of the 70's and beginning of 80's.[4,5] In these years the interest for animal cognition, intelligence, consciousness passions and emotions has flourished (interested readers can refer to "Minding animal"[6] written by canine expert and bioethicist Mark Bekoff) as well as it has increased the interest for the ways in which humans interact and communicate with species with which they have the closest contact and vice versa.

The ability to communicate in the absence of a common articulate language and to modify their emotions in a reciprocal way is an essential and founding element for the ability of dogs to act as therapists. The first scientific record of such ability dates back to the 70's, when, in the laboratory of Harry Harlow at the University of Wisconsin and in the California Primate Center directed by Bill Mason at Davis, highly original research was conducted on primates in the field of ethology and psychobiology, in order to identify the selective features characterizing the relationship which is established early on between a newborn and its mother. This research was highly revolutionary for that time. It highlighted the basic role played by the mother-infant relationship (in which both members have a reciprocal "creative" and "active" role) in shaping the emotional behaviour of the offspring. Moreover, these studies shed light on the possible mechanisms underlying the vulnerability and onset of psychiatric disorders, such as autism, and, especially, the possible outcome on neuropsychological development resulting from malfunctional bonding created during the neonatal and infantile phases. In these studies, young conspecifics (monkey therapists, characterised by an adolescent phase with a strong filial bond) were used for the recovery of juvenile monkeys with autistic characteristics. It was of interest that other species, dogs in particular, would found to be effective, while inanimate surrogates (cloth-covered plastic horse) would not.[7–10]

Recent studies on humans have shown that a relationship with an animal, not exclusively a dog, can ameliorate the self-confidence and increase the learning capabilities and the motivation to interact socially.

What Is Pet Therapy

The term "pet therapy" was coined in 1964 after a child psychiatrist Boris M. Levinson, observed positive effects while using his dog, Jingles, in sessions with severely withdrawn children. He noticed that the dog served as an ice-breaker and provided a focus for communication. Thanks to the animal, Levinson was able to establish a relationship with the child and start an effective therapy. Since then, scientists and health professionals have put Levinson's theories into practice and now a wide range of health professionals recognize what many pet owners have known for years–i.e. that pets can be good for our health and well-being.

It is important to notice that nowadays professionals discourage the term "pet therapy" because it actually refers to animal behaviour training programs and prefer to distinguish between:

- *Animal Assisted Activities* (AAA) provide opportunities for motivational, educational, and/or recreational benefits in order to enhance quality of life of some human categories such as blind and physical or psychic handicapped persons. AAA are delivered in a variety of environments by specially trained professionals, para-professionals, and/or volunteers in association with animals that meet specific criteria.
- *Animal Assisted Therapies* (AAT) are goal-directed interventions in which an animal meeting specific criteria is an integral part of the treatment process. AAT are delivered and/or directed by a health/human service provider working within the scope of his or her profession. AAT are designed to promote improvement in human physical, social, emotional, and/or cognitive functioning. They are provided in a variety of settings and may involve groups or be individual in nature. This process is documented and evaluated.

In Italy pet therapy has been recognized as official care by a Legislative Decree (DL.vo issued on February 28th 2003; following an agreement between the State and the Italian Regions). For the first time in our country, this Decree sanctioned the role that an animal could have in the emotional life of a person and the therapeutic benefits derived from pet animals.

Who can Benefit from Pet Therapy

People who usually can benefit from pet therapy are:

Children

Pet therapy decreases children's stress and anxiety about illness, injury and hospital experience. Interacting with a pet can sometimes enhance recovery following a serious illness. It can change behaviour, create a sense of responsibility and even improve a child's ability to participate in therapeutic treatment leading to attainment identified goals and objectives. Children are often extremely trusting and easily achieve a level of intimacy with animals. This special bond contributes to pets' effectiveness as co-therapists.[11]

Elderly persons

In the institutionalized elderly there is evidence that pet therapy may reduce depression, blood pressure, irritability and agitation, and may increase social interaction. In an epidemiological study performed on people that had suffered from infarction, the presence of a pet was found to have a positive effect on survival.[12] In Alzheimer's disease there is evidence that the presence of a companion animal may increase social behaviours such as smiles, laughs, looks, leans, touches, verbalizations, name-calling, or others. Moreover pet therapy has been shown to reduce loneliness and depression in residents of long-term care facilities, particularly in people with a prior history of pet ownership. The presence of a pet has also been found to lead to increased verbal interactions among residents.[13]

Psychiatric patients

There is evidence that presence of a pet among psychiatric patients promotes social interactions.[14] In people with schizophrenia pet therapy may lead to improved interest in rewarding activities as well as better use of leisure time and improved motivation. There is also evidence of improvement in socialization skills, independent living, and general well-being. In a large, well-designed study, hospitalized patients with a variety of psychiatric disorders were found to have reduced anxiety after a single session of Pet therapy for most, the benefits were superior to those of a session of regular recreation therapy.

Educational Activities Promoted by Pet Relationships

According to some reports, pets, with their morphological and behavioural diversity, could solicit the child in the formation and enrichment of its imaginary world, offering him/her more than one model for his/her elaborative processes and strengthening his/her imagination. Moreover, the interaction with the animal diversity, or the simple referring to it, could help the child in coping with a multifaceted world, transforming the diffidence in curiosity and tolerance and decreasing widespread fear. The act of taking care of a companion animal usually decreases generally aggressive behaviours, negligence, little helpfulness. Pet relationships increase affectivity, fortify the epimeletic tendency of a child, the capabilities to take care, to help and protect someone, and decrease general disorganization, low attention to external and inner world. Moreover, this relationship helps a young boy/girl in having a positive behaviour in all the daily activities.

Usually, pets have juvenile characteristics able to stimulate communication and to solicit children to play activities. Pet owners taking care of their animals, give rise to an epimeletic behaviour and children observing this situation carry out an identification process by which they come to play the role of an adult. The "encounter" with the animal can be of great help in shaping the emotional ability of the child. This can be achieved because the relationship with the animal has an emotional and empathic connotation and eventually leads the child to learn how to self-regulate its arousal states, in order to effectively interact with the pet.

An increasing motivation and attention has been observed, for example, when pets are regularly in school classes in which children with mental retardation are present. Pet became the centre of attraction ameliorating, at least in part, the learning capability deficits of these children. It is well known the study on an autistic girl that learned to count up to three just to start a game in which her dog was involved in.

Animals Used as Pet Therapists
The animals most commonly used for pet therapy are:

Dog

This is, by large, the most frequently used animal as co-therapist, both with children, adults and elderly people. By soliciting play, dogs arouse patients and demand interactions, in addition to offering company.

Cat

It is enrolled as co-therapist for its independence and the easy way to take care of it. It is preferred by people living alone or having an age or some pathologies that limit their movements.[15]

Hamster and rabbit

To observe, to pet and to take care of these animals could bring great benefits, especially to children having a hard time in their life.

Horse

Horses are mostly employed for medical, rehabilitative and psychological-educative hippotherapy practised in equipped facilities by the help of a well trained staff. Autistic children, Down syndrome children, disabled persons with behavioural and motor dysfunctions can benefit from hippotherapy.

Bird

Studies performed on groups of elderly people have evidenced the beneficial effects of the usually taking care of birds, in particular parrots.

Fish

It has been noticed that the observation of a fish in an aquarium might help in reducing tachycardia and muscles strain, acting as an anti-stress.

Dolphin

These animals have been employment as co-therapists in the case of depression and mental and emotional disorders. The dolphin therapy can improve autistic patients' psychological status and social adaptation.

Donkey, Goat and Cow

These are domestic animals that can also be employed in pet therapy practises.

By and large, domestic animals, particularly small mammals, should be preferred as Pet Therapists as they are those that have been selected for their ability to interact socially (and emotionally) with humans.

Professional Categories Involved in Pet Therapy: The Working Group

In Pet therapy, the activity performed by the "animal therapist" towards the "human patient" is very complex and to be successful, above all, it requires the contribution of many professional figures.

For this reason, every Pet therapy experience is the results of the combined effort of a cross-disciplinary team made up of various professional categories. These categories interact and bring their own specific contribution in a complementary way.

As operators, the members of the team work personally at the design, at the evaluation of programs and at the execution of activities and therapies. In particular, it is important that these activities do not result stressful for the animal itself.[16]

Ideally, the Pet therapy team should be made of all (or most) of the following figures:

Physician
Psychiatrist
Psychologist
Rehabilitation therapist
Social worker
Nurse
Teacher
Pedagogue
Vet
Ethnologist
Professional dog trainer
Pet conductor

Pilot Study on AAA and AAT Activities in a Sample Region of Italy: Emilia Romagna

The increasing interest in pet therapy and the lack of guidelines that formally regulate the therapies performed with animals, has raised the need to document the activities that are being undertaken in Italy under this label. This initiative involves the Istituto Superiore di Sanità and the Faculty of Veterinary Medicine of the University of Bologna, and is aimed to chart all the initiatives in this field in continuous expansion, in the Italian region Emilia Romagna.

The goal of our study was to identify both the common and the discriminating factors between several operators recognised in the Emilia Romagna territory and to collect them in macro-groups of "certification". To this purpose we selectively identified a number of parameters, such as the professional profile of pet operators, the formative background of animals employed, the typology of users, the type and the degree of the handicap, the type of structure in which the activities are performed and the institutions involved.

A first consideration on the professional profile of the operators brings out the fact that in the region Emilia Romagna the majority of people belonging to this category has the *Referee Pet Operator* certificate or the *Pet Partner Operator* certificate, qualifications obtained after attending the *Referee in Welfare Zooanthropology* course organized by the SIUA (Scuola di interazione uomo-animale: Man Animal Interaction School). A smaller group of operators in Emilia Romagna has an AIUCA (Associazione Italiana Uso Cani d'Assistenza: Italian Association Use of Dog for Assistance) certificate and performs activities with equine horse therapists. Finally, an additional group enlists an operator having a Delta Society certificate who interacts with veterinarians (Figure 1).

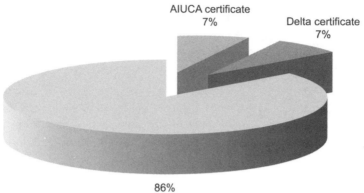

AIUCA certificate
7%

Delta certificate
7%

86%
SIUA certificate

Figure 1. Professional certification of pet therapy operators.

Pet operators, for the most part, are graduates in Pedagogy, Veterinary Medicine, Psychology, Environmental Sciences, Natural Sciences, Medicine, Biological Sciences, Pharmacy, Geology, or high school diploma, Dog trainer, operators in social services, hold Diplomas for Athletic/Physical trainer (Figure 2).

Many projects of AAA and of AAT are listed as zooanthropology projects for children (Zooantropologia Didattica, ZD). These are projects of Pet Education devoted to children aged 2-16, some with handicap of different types. These operators, in addition to the certificates in *Referee in Welfare Zooanthropology* or *Certified Pet Partner Couple*, also obtained a certificate in *Referee in Didactic Zooanthropology* at the SIUA or by SCIVAC (Società Culturale Italiana Veterinari per Animali da Compagnia: Italian Cultural Society of Companion Animal Vets) (Figure 3).

In some cases the operators with a certificate in *Certified Pet Partner Couple* and *Referee in Welfare Zooanthropology* are also *Dog Educators*, certificate obtained at the SIUA.

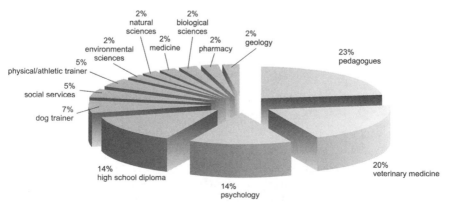

2%
natural
sciences

2%
biological
sciences

2%
environmental
sciences

2%
medicine

2%
pharmacy

2%
geology

23%
pedagogues

5%
physical/athletic trainer

5%
social services

7%
dog trainer

14%
high school diploma

14%
psychology

20%
veterinary medicine

Figure 2. Education/main occupation of pet therapy operators.

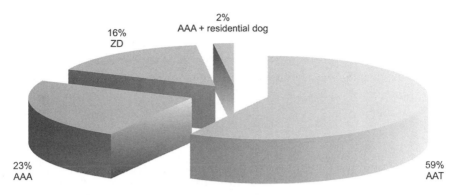

Figure 3. Relative occurrence of AAT/AAA projects (in Emilia Romagna 26 ZD projects have been reported).

As for training courses involving dogs, subjects coming from amateur farms, but also dogs coming from kennels and professional farms have attended the *Certified Pet Partner Couple* Course. Following this training, dogs obtain the SIUA certification for A, B, C, D category.

On the other hand, to become *Referee Pet Operator*, the dog has to attend a course of *Basic Education* and of *Education to Relationship*. This allows it to take part in a working group (without forming a certificated couple).

One case of *Certification of Dog for Assistance and Therapy* has been documented at the *Assistance Dog Institute*, Rounert Park, California and one dog was found certified by *Delta Society*.

Sporadically, animals belonging to various species such as dwarf rabbits, California rabbits, dwarf Tibetan goats (coming from farms unharmed from brucellosis), cats, turtles and tortoise have been reported as being used as pet therapists (Figure 4).

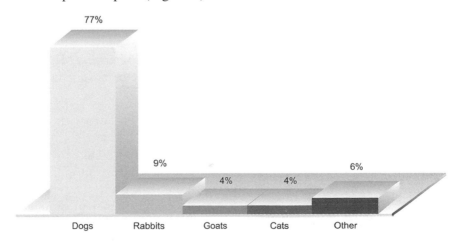

Figure 4. Animals usually used as pet therapists.

The typology of AAA and AAT users is represented, mostly, by children and elderly, followed by adolescents and adults. As for children, there are subjects with verified diagnosis of hyperactivity, deficits in learning, Down syndrome, West syndrome, Rett syndrome, mental delay, speech and communication disorders of different levels (degree), as well hospitalized children.

As for adolescent, these are teens with physical and/or psychic handicap, experiencing social unease and maladjustment.

Adults are psychiatric patients with schizophrenic symptoms and relational disorders, in addition to cases of autism, psychosis, mental handicap, premature senile dementia and mental retardation. Carriers of psychiatric pathologies associated with cognitive deficits as well patients in semi vegetative status due to severe brain lesions, patients with post-traumatic psycho-physic disabilities, ex drug abusers with confused and depressive states.

In the case of elderly people, the pathologies more often found are senile dementia, Alzheimer's disease, confused and anxious states, mental and physic disabilities, motor disorders.

The structures hosting pet therapy projects are public structures such as nursery schools, kindergarten schools, elementary schools, middle schools, high schools, residential homes for adolescents without family, residential houses, daytime centres for disabled, institutes of public assistance and charities (socio-rehabilitative daytime centres and sheltered houses for elderly), the Judicial Psychiatric Hospital of Reggio Emilia. Between the private structures we can enlist: nursery schools, private structures for disabled people, private houses with children and adolescents. Hospital structures in which pet therapy is performed are: the Judicial Psychiatric Hospital of Reggio Emilia, and the Paediatric ward "Gozzadini" of the S. Orsola Hospital of Bologna. In some other Hospitals, such as the Rizzoli Hospital of Bologna and "The house of Awakenings Luca De Nigris" (Department of Neurosciences, Maggiore Hospital and Bellaria Hospital), AAT projects have been scheduled to start but have not yet been activated (Figure 5, Figure 6).

The institutions involved included numerous towns with surroundings and villages–Bologna (Calderara di Reno, Casalecchio di Reno, Castel San Pietro, Granarolo dell'Emilia, Osteria Grande, San Giorgio di Piano, San Giovanni in Persiceto, Zola Predosa), Modena (Castelfranco Emilia, Carpi, Castelnuovo Rangone, Campogalliano, Formigine, Sassuolo), Reggio Emilia (Bagnolo in Piano), Ravenna –, the Province of Bologna, the Region Emilia Romagna, the Office for Animals Rights of Bologna, The Society of Transport of Ravenna, the Faculty of Pedagogy of the

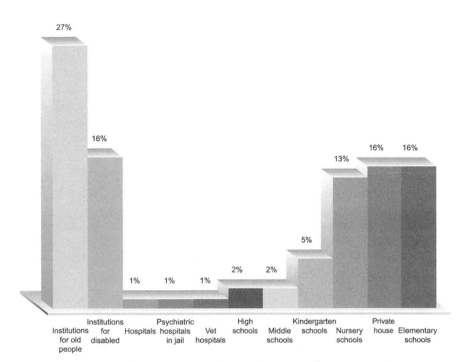

Figure 5. Main structures hosting AAA and AAT activities.

University of Bologna, the Institute Charitas of Modena, some social cooperatives, the Local Health Unit of Modena, the Services of Paediatric Neuropsychiatry of the Local Health Unit of Modena.

In the region Emilia Romagna, from 2001 to 2006 included, 37 AAA projects were registered as well as 92 AAT projects, 26 zooanthropology projects for children and adults, 3 AAA projects (one is still ongoing) forecasting the permanent custody of the dog to the structure in which the activities are performed.

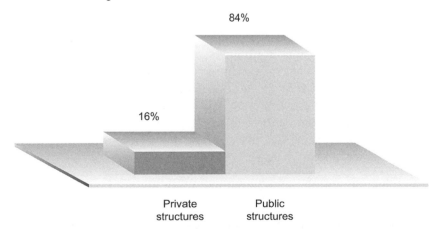

Figure 6. Main structures hosting AAA and AAT activities.

Forty-one operators have been involved: 37 work for 7 groups registered and 4 work as individuals. The total number of animals involved is greater than the one of the animals really used in the projects carried out. However, 56 animals overall were used, 43 of which were dogs. In relation to the institutions involved in the project from 2001 to 2006, 26 are institution for the elderly, 15 institutions for adolescent disabled, 14 elementary schools, 11 nursery schools, 5 kindergarten, 2 middle schools, 2 high schools, 1 private nursery school, 1 nursery school breast-fed section, a veterinary surgery of Local Health Unit at the municipal kennel, 1 judicial psychiatric hospital, 1 general hospital, 14 private houses (Figure 5).

The smallest number estimated of users profiting by services delivered between 2001 and 2006 (excluding projects devoted to primary and nursery schools for which it could be too arbitrary to establish a minimum number of users) reaches the number of 407.

Conclusions

Overall, Pet therapy and AAA have revealed, with time, their potential ability to heal as well as to provide opportunities to enhance the quality of the life of people with physical and mental disabilities.[17]

At the institutional level, growing efforts have raised attention in pet therapy and AAA. However, no established methodologies are presently available for the therapeutic exploitation of animals, but the pressing need to help affected categories, especially children, has stimulated scattered efforts at an explosive pace.

The Istituto Superiore di Sanità, which plays an important advisory role in the Italian health system, has being taking an ever increasing role in attempting to regulate these activities by e.g. selecting good-quality training activities at the public academic system level (mainly University courses and Masters) and by sponsoring a few pilot experiences.

In this rapidly growing field, we are attempting to fill the need for (i) identifying standard curriculum for trainers, avoiding spontaneous initiatives; (ii) establishing, by means of a scientific consensus (both at the European and national level) a draft of guidelines to be implemented in the near future in selected centers, endowed by good scientific and clinical credentials; (iii) promoting, at the international level, university research in pet/ humans relationships, in order to study how dog's emotions are communicated to humans and other dogs.

Notes

1. Serpell J. *In the company of animals—A study of human-animal relationships*. Canto edition published ed: Cambridge University Press; 1996.
2. Coren S. *Capire il linguaggio dei cani*. Roma: Franco Muzio; 2003.

3. Hare B, Brown M, Williamson C, Tomasello M. The domestication of social cognition in dogs. *Science* 2002; 298(5598):1634–1636.

4. Ristau CA. (Ed). *Cognitive ethology: The minds of other animals. essays in honor of Donald R. Griffin.* Hillsdale (New Jersey): Lawrence Erlabaum Associates; 1991.

5. Griffin DR. *The question of animal awareness—Evolutionary continuity of mental experience.* New York: The Rockefeller University Press; 1976.

6. Bekoff M. *Minding animals: awareness, emotions, and heart.* Oxford: Oxford University Press; 2002.

7. Mason WA, Kenney MD. Redirection of filial attachments in Rhesus Monkeys: Dogs as mother surrogates. *Science* 1974; 183:1209–1211.

8. Redefer LA, Goodman JF. Pet facilitated therapy with autistic children. *Journal of Autism and Development* 1989;19: 461–467.

9. McNicholas J, Collis GM. Relationships between young people with autism and their Pets. In: *7th International conference on human-animal interactions: animals, health and the quality of life.* Geneva; 6–9 September 1995.

10. Davis H, Balafur D. (Ed). *The inevitable bond. Examining scientist-animal interactions*: Cambridge University Press; 1992.

11. Marchesini R. *Fondamenti di zooantropologia <<z- Zooantropologia applicata.* Bologna: Alberto Perdisa (Airplane S.r.l.); 2005.

12. Friedman E, Katcher A, Lynch JJ, Thomas SA. Animal companions and one-year survival of patients after discharge from a coronary care unit. *Public Health Reports* 1980; 95: 307–312.

13. Corson SA, Corson EOL, Learly E, Gwynne PH, Arnold LE. Pet facilitated psychotherapy in a hospital setting. *Current Psychiatric Therapies* 1975; 15: 277–286.

14. Barker SB, Dawson KS. The effects of animal-assisted therapy on anxiety ratings of hospitalized psychiatric patients. *Psychiatr Serv* 1998; 49(6):797–801.

15. Turner DC, Bateson P. (Ed). *The Domestic Cat. The biology of its behaviour*: Cambridge University Press; 2000.

16. Nagel M, v. Reinhardt C. *Lo stress nel cane.* Cormano (MI): Haquihna; 2003.

17. Cirulli F, Natoli E, Alleva E. Utilizzo di un corretto rapporto uomo animale ai fini di una riabilitazione psicologica: la Pet therapy in Italia. In: *Atti del Seminario "Recenti tematiche in biologia e medicina: dalla ricerca scientifica un sostegno alle persone disabili".* Istituto Superiore di Sanità, Roma; 23 marzo 1998.

DOCUMENT 11: THE MORAL BASIS OF ANIMAL-ASSISTED THERAPY—TZACHI ZAMIR*

Society & Animals 14:2 (2006) © Koninklijke Brill NV, Leiden, 2006.
Reprinted by permission of the Animals and Society Institute, Inc.

Abstract

Is nonhuman animal-assisted therapy (AAT) a form of exploitation? After exploring possible moral vindications of AAT and after establishing a distinction between "use" and "exploitation," the essay distinguishes

*Tzachi Zamir, The Hebrew University, Jerusalem

between forms of animal-assisted therapy that are morally unobjectionable and those modes of it that ought to be abolished.

Nonhuman animal-assisted therapy (AAT)[1] is becoming increasingly popular. Expositors claim that its roots go back to the eighteenth century when Tuke, one of the originators of modern psychiatry, introduced its use in his work with his patients. Nowadays, AAT encompasses interventions incorporating dogs, cats, rodents, birds, reptiles, horses, monkeys, and even dolphins. The goals of such therapy are extremely varied, including psychological, therapeutic objectives as well as other forms of assistance.[2]

In this essay, I will ignore the prudential questions that plague almost all AAT literature that I have come across; that is, whether the benefits of AAT can be shown conclusively over and against more conventional modes of therapy. I will assume—what is in fact highly controversial—that AAT is therapeutically effective generally and, for some individuals, is advantageous when compared with other forms of therapy. Can such uses of nonhuman animals be morally justified from a "liberationist" perspective, a perspective that acknowledges that animals are not merely a resource to be exploited by humans?[3] Practitioners of AAT often say that they work with animals rather than "use" them. The primary distinction that this essay formulates is the one between use and exploitation. I then pursue the implications of this distinction to the moral status of AAT.

The Case Against AAT

AAT literature does not ignore the moral dimension of the work that it advocates. Yet the remarks on ethics appear to be limited to considerations of welfare. The *Delta Society*'s website, for example, warns its readers that AAT may be inappropriate for the animals when:

1. injuries from rough handling or from other animals may occur;
2. basic animal welfare cannot be assured (this includes veterinary care and access to water and exercise areas; and
3. the animal does not enjoy visiting.

In a different publication by the same organization, it is maintained that "At all times the rights of the animals shall be respected and ensured. This includes humane treatment, protection from undue stress, and availability of water and exercise area" (Grammonley et al., 1997, p. 2). One proposed code of ethics for animal-assisted therapy includes requirements:

1. The animal's welfare must be the priority of the therapy facilitator;
2. The therapy animal must "never be forced to leave the home to go to work" or to perform actions that it is reluctant to perform; and
3. Animals are to be given adjustment time and quiet time periods before sessions and be protected from individuals carrying diseases that may be transmitted to them. (Preziosi, 1997, pp. 5–6)

Yet from a broader liberationist perspective, such remarks barely scratch the surface of the moral questions that AAT raises. A liberationist stance ascribes value not only to the life of the animal but also to the quality of such a life— as well as to the value of the animal's freedom—in the sense that lack of freedom requires a moral justification. For liberationists, using animals to treat humans is potentially immoral in six distinct ways:

Limitations of Freedom

Companion animals need to be kept by the therapists or be temporary companion animals of the individual being treated. In some cases, when the animals are in effect modified pets (like guide dogs), the limitations of freedom are the same as those involved in all pet-owner relationships (relationships that are themselves immoral for some liberationists, regardless of their quality). In the case of animals who are not pets or modified pets (rabbits, hamsters, chinchillas, snakes, birds, all of whom respond to human beings but, unlike alarm or service dogs, do not appear to derive pleasure from such interaction and seem incapable of transferring their social needs onto humans), the loss of freedom may be much more severe.

Life Determination

Freedom can be curtailed for a temporary period (confining a wounded animal in the wild and then releasing the animal once the animal has healed). But unlike limitation-of-freedom actions, some actions with regard to animals are total and life-determining. Turning an animal into a companion animal, into an animal in the zoo, into a race horse, a jumper, or an event horse are life-determining actions. The decision to employ an animal therapeutically involves making such a total decision regarding a particular animal.

Training

Getting dogs or monkeys to assist humans efficiently in numerous tasks involves a prolonged period of training, which itself includes various violations of the animal's well being. Creating horses for therapy (therapy-horses) requires "breaking" them. Moreover, unlike cats and dogs, many of the other animals used in AAT are frightened by human presence, and they have to undergo periods in which they get accustomed to humans around them.

Social Disconnection

Simians live in packs. By turning them into nursing entities, one disconnects them from whatever it is that they maintain through their social context. The same holds for rabbits or other rodents who are isolated from their kin. There is, to be sure, a certain degree of mystery here both regarding the nature of the social needs and the way they might be internally experienced as a loss by the animal. Yet it is morally safe to make the probable assumption that such disconnection (or bringing up the animal without contact with the animal's kin) is a form of deprivation.

Injury

Animals for therapy (therapy-animals) can be (and are) routinely manhandled. Even when gently handled, exposing them to strangers who pet them can itself create anxieties in them. A small percentage of such animals are injured during these sessions.[4]

Instrumentalization

Liberationists tend to tacitly or explicitly model ideal human-nonhuman relations on analogies with human-human ethics. While few extend to animals— the same range of moral considerability that befits humans— liberationists turn the human-non human model from the thoughtless instrumentalization that is typical of human relations with objects into forms of interaction that approximate human-human relations. From this perspective, since it is unimaginable to retain a sub-group of human beings as therapeutic aids of other human beings even if proved as facilitating extremely effective therapy (say that the tactile quality of touching members of this subgroup is proved to have therapeutic merits), doing this to animals is wrong in a similar way. Animals are not out there to be used, even when the use is important or worthy.

Liberationists would be quick to identify these six potential violations of the moral status of animals and would accordingly be concerned about the moral legitimacy of AAT as such. The fact that much more serious violations than the six noted above occur does not abrogate the moral questions that relate to the six violations. It matters not that billions of animals are routinely killed for negligible reasons or that they are institutionally used and exploited in large-scale industries all over the world. If these six violations cannot be vindicated, liberationists should censor these modalities of therapy and assistance.

A Paternalistic Case for AAT?

Analyzing the moral status of the six potential violations invites an exploration of the pet-owner relationship. If pet-owner relationships can be morally justified, some of the therapeutic uses of animals sketched above might be vindicated as well.[5] I have elsewhere proposed a utilitarian-based justification of the pet-owner relationship that can morally legitimate the practice of keeping some animals as pets. In a nutshell, my claim was that the handsoff approach advocated by some liberationists—the idea that the lives of animals are better the less paternalistic they are—is morally sound though, ironically, not always in the interest of the animals themselves. Accordingly, I urged liberationists to avoid the hands-off approach.[6] With regard to companion animals, some pet-owner relationships are an overall good for human as well as for nonhuman animals. The paternalistic framework of such relations is a potential wrong but is exonerated because it makes for a better world for small animals: It is an overall better alternative for them than a life in the wild. Success stories of feral populations of horses and dogs would modify such an impression only in few examples but are less impressive when thinking about highly populated countries in which such animals would turn into "pests" and would be treated accordingly. Cats and dogs get to lead longer, safer, and more comfortable lives. While they lose through this exchange too (loss of freedom, being subjected to various operative interventions), such losses are offset by the benefits to them in the long run (limiting movement can prolong the life of the pet since it diminishes the risks of accidents and injury from fighting other animals—a neutered animal lives longer).[7]

In other cases, such losses help preserve the pet-owner relations as such (most owners would refuse to keep animals who can freely reproduce), relations the existence of which is an overall good for the pets. Such welfare-based thinking can also generate welfare-based distinctions that can tell us when pet abuse takes place and can guide some moral decision-making within small animal veterinary medicine. Some paternalistic, invasive, owner actions are justified on welfare ground, as the overall good for companion animals trumps their inability to understand the action (vaccination). Other such actions are obviously immoral, as they do not promote any animal interest and advance a marginal interest of the owner (ear docking). Most other actions fall in the middle and should be assessed in terms of the overall good for the animal, the owner, and in terms of available alternatives to the examined action.

For some animals, turning them into companion animals is not a benefit to them in any obvious way (wild animals and birds); so, welfare considerations urge us to banish the attempt to keep such animals as pets. Yet the same considerations suggest that the practice of keeping companion animals is not objectionable as such: An ideal liberationist world will include pet-owner relationships, and such relations—at their best—also show us that a paternalistic, yet non-exploitative, human-animal relation is both possible and actual.

Can animal-therapy be justified in a similar way? "Service" animals such as signal and guide dogs easily fall into the pet-owner category; so, such practices are, in principle, justified. Dogs do pay a price for such lives: They are spayed or neutered, trained for long periods (in the case of guide dogs much longer than other dogs), and isolated from their kin. But dogs seem to be able to transfer their social needs onto humans, and some of the prolonged training can arguably be an advantage, providing important (and pleasurable) mental stimulation to these dogs. If humanity were to endorse a handsoff approach with regard to animals, such dogs would appear to lead qualitatively inferior (and probably shorter) lives in the wild—even in the few countries in the world in which the notion of "the wild" still makes sense.

Some AAT programs strive to connect animal interests and human needs by placing shelter-abandoned animals with elderly people, thus benefiting particular animals in an even more immediate way.[8] Is a capuchin monkey, captured in the wild, isolated from the pack, trained using electric shocks, had teeth extracted—all of these prior to placing the monkey as a nurse of a handicapped person, better off than living in the wild?[9] The answer is here negative. Such an animal is better off having nothing to do with humans. In such examples, the hands-off approach is not only morally sound but is also continuous with the animal's welfare. The same holds for other forms of AAT: Maintaining stressed rodents in petting areas in educational and therapeutic institutions for the projected benefit of children, psychiatric patients, or prisoners who may enjoy various therapeutic benefits through this connection does not appear to promote any of the rodent's own interests.[10] The lives of these rodents apart from humans appear to be a better alternative for them.

The same considerations help make sense of horse-assisted therapy. Justifying hippotherapy brings up the range of moral issues relating to equine husbandry and the moral status of the diverse practices it involves (racing, show jumping, hunting, riding as such). Horses require lengthy training periods and demand the use of bits and harnesses. Many of them are then kept in very small locks. They are subjected to all of the medical interventions that cats and dogs undergo. All of these practices would disturb liberationists. Yet where and how would horses exist in an ideal liberationist world? Reserves might be an option in some countries in which feral populations of horses might be feasible. But in many parts of the world, a puritanical decision to let horses be would boil down to a horseless environment.

Liberationists would know that the argument from the animal's projected welfare is a risky one to make, since the idea that the animal's existence justifies exploiting the animal is routinely used in various forms, supposedly vindicating all kinds of animal abuse. However, I believe that in the context of AAT this justification is viable.[11] I do, however, wish to add that since equine husbandry appears to be economically driven through and through, the idea that some relations between humans and horses are justified in the sense that they ultimately benefit horses does not morally cleanse all such relationships. It is not obvious to me that practices such as racing, dressage, or show jumping are morally justified, as they involve pain and risk of injury to the animal, and—according to one veterinarian I have consulted, Orit Zamir DVM—they can radically curtail the life-span of the horses and diminish its quality. Hippotherapy, by contrast, is not a form of human-animal connection that appears detrimental to the horse. The utilitarian benefits for such horses—they get to exist,[12] lead safe and relatively comfortable lives, are not abused or exploited—outweigh the prices they pay.

Use Versus Exploitation

I have so far argued that for some animals AAT cannot be vindicated through appeals to the overall good for the animal through the animal's forced participation in a paternalistic relationship with humans. Could some other framework justify using animals for therapeutic purposes? In this section, I will discuss (and reject) two such possible justifications: Cartesianism and Kantianism. Later in this essay, I address Utilitarianism and Speciesism.

Cartesians claim that animals lack moral considerability. For a Cartesian, it is senseless to draw a morally relevant distinction between animals and objects (for Descartes, this also involved a denial of animal pain). Since animals lack moral considerability, any action done to them—AAT included— is morally permissible. Kantians are fig-leaf Cartesians. They agree with Cartesians that animals lack any kind of intrinsic moral status. But they also claim that some actions with respect to animals are morally reprehensible. This stems not from anything having to do with the animal but from how such actions determine the agents that performed them:—from what these actions say about them or about humanity in general. Cartesians would have no problem with any form of AAT since, for them, animals are no more than means to an end. Kantians would concur with this, adding the restriction that no abuse or cruelty should take place as part of AAT (consistent Cartesians would have no problem with cruelty to therapy animals, if it is shown to be therapeutically beneficial to human patients.)[13]

The more general issue of the moral considerability of animals cannot be broached here. Liberationists have offered detailed criticisms of the Cartesian and Kantian frameworks. My own arguments against these positions, as well as my own position regarding the moral considerability of animals as such, is available elsewhere.[14] In our context, both positions constitute a theoretical, not a practical, opposition. By this, I mean that judging by the literature that they produce and by their concern with animal welfare, people involved in offering AAT appear to be both sensitive and concerned about the well being of the animals on whom they rely. They would find it odd to think that one may do anything one likes to an animal (Cartesianism) or that torturing a dog is wrong, not because of the dog but only because of what this says about the torturer (Kantianism).[15]

Short of a categorical denial of moral status, AAT advocates may favor weaker forms of these positions. They might try to defend the idea that using animals is permissible, even when detrimental to their welfare, so long as no abuse takes place. They will argue that such use does not constitute exploitation. The liberationism I have outlined above, in which some instrumental human animal relations are morally legitimate, although they constitute a use of animals, is close to this position—but importantly different not only in general moral categories but also in terms of the consequences for particular species in the context of AAT.

To palpably perceive this difference, we need to draw some distinctions regarding instrumentalization. We now approach the conceptual heart of this essay: the distinction between use and exploitation and the manner by which this distinction affects the moral status (or lack of it) of AAT.

Actual practice pressurizes those who would like to relate to avoiding instrumentalization as a morally meaningful value. We routinely use our friends and relations for emotional or physical support. We use other people for their abilities, knowledge, and work power. And since give-and-take relations are a legitimate part of life, the relevant moral distinction is not the one between instrumentalization and non-instrumentalization but the one between use and exploitation. Kant was unhelpful regarding this, holding that whereas in some contexts it is permissible to treat another person as a means, it is immoral to perceive another person *merely* as a means. This position is notoriously vague, since it appeals to private motivations that are easily given to manipulation and rationalization. People can and do exploit others while commending themselves for negligible concessions that they make for the benefit of the exploited party.

Fortunately, the distinction between use and exploitation is not hard to draw. X uses Y when X perceives Y as a means of furthering X's own financial (or other) well being. This turns into exploitation when X is willing to act in a way that is substantially detrimental to Y's own well being in order to further X's own. By "substantial," I mean that the action predictably carries consequences such as shortening Y's life, damaging Y's health, limiting Y's freedom, abusing what Y is (some forms of prostitution), systematically thwarting Y's potential (child labor), and subjecting Y to pain or to a strongly undesired life (demanding inhuman workloads and thus creating human-slavery). In addition, exploitation usually suggests lack of consent by the exploited party (or a consent predicated on a highly limited choice or on choosing among impossible alternatives). Exploitation is also mostly related to the existence of unequal power-relations or some dependency relations between the parties, favoring the exploiting party in an institutional and systematic way.

To know for certain that X is not exploiting Y, merely using Y, X must repeatedly make choices that substantively further Y's welfare even when in conflict with X's own prudential motives. This need not mean that X is to become irrational or altruistic. It merely suggests how persons can actually verify that they are not involved in an exploitative relationship. I believe that people can legitimately fall short of this ideal. That is, they can be uncertain as to whether a particular relationship that they have is exploitative. Give-and take relations can be vague in this sense. For example, immigrants in welloff countries sometimes offer to overwork themselves so as to provide for the families in their home countries. Fantasizing about global justice is nice as a thought-experiment, but it does not help one when compelled to choose between cooperating with such requests or not. One does not always know. And provided that one does not knowingly participate in, or cooperate with, clear-cut exploitative relations, I believe that it is morally permissible to have relations over which one has some misgivings.

How can one tell whether one is in a "clear-cut" exploitative relationship? Generally, you are exploiting an entity if your relationship with it predictably benefits you and harms the entity. More specifically and in light of the various characterizations of exploitative relationships mentioned above, the answer is both quantitative and qualitative: Relationships become more exploitative if they share more of the characteristics spelled out above (this is the "quantitative" answer). At the same time, a relationship can manifest only one of the characteristics mentioned above in some substantial way and be clearly exploitative (the "qualitative" answer). If, for example, I provide an entity with a comfortable life in which it is not abused in any way yet aim to kill it when it is very young the relationship is clearly exploitative. If, on the other hand, I intend to terminate the entity's life only if it becomes old or incurably ill, I am not exploiting it, even if I would not act in the same way with regard to a human being. This is why pet-owner relationships can be non-exploitative (although they might constitute use) and why the same cannot be said concerning the lamb industry. I am not claiming that distinguishing between use and exploitation is always simple. Indeed, animalethics provide many vague cases (free roaming, de-beaked hens, for instance). But the considerations that could lead us in deciding these issues are not mysterious and many times indicate decisive answers.

We are now in a position to assess the modified Cartesian/Kantian counterargument to my proposal. I have argued that animals may be used

but may not be exploited and have tried to unpack this distinction. Applied
to AAT, this means that service dogs are used, though not exploited, since
their welfare is promoted by the relationship. Horses too gain much from
their relations with humans. The same cannot be said for rodents, snakes,
birds, aquarium-kept dolphins, or monkeys who gain little or nothing
through AAT and lose a lot.[16] Unlike horses or dogs, all of these creatures
can easily exist in the wild in large numbers; by turning them into vehicles
for therapy, both their freedom and their social needs are radically curtailed. Counter to my opponent's claims, AAT that uses these creatures
is exploitative, even if no abuse takes place.

Two Objections

Before examining whether exploiting animals can be defended as such,
I need to respond to two counterarguments to what I have just said. The
first is that I am downplaying the significance of the price horses and dogs
pay for their existence in the company of humans. Watching a horse
struggle with the bit in his mouth is a difficult sight. "Breaking" horses or
the prolonged training periods that service dogs undergo can boil down
to painful activities and deprivation, especially when the training system
is not (or is not only) reward-based. Moreover, the import of thwarting
the procreative potential of these animals by neutering them cannot be
ignored.

The second objection has to do with the argument from non-existence on
which I relied when claiming that dogs and horses gain from their relations with humans, since this relationship means that they exist. I have
said that I defend the metaphysical plausibility of such an argument elsewhere. In a nutshell, I argue that a non-existent entity cannot be harmed
by not bringing "it" into existence, yet it—now without the quotes—can
benefit from a decision to bring it into existence. There is nothing contra-
dictory about an entity having both these properties. But there is a non-
metaphysically based objection to this move having to do with species
as opposed to particular entities. I have said that, in most countries, horses
and dogs are not likely to exist outside of use-based human relations and
that abrogating all such relations will, in any case, imply a radical reduction in the number of such beings. But an AAT therapist can choose to
breed particular rodents for the purpose of using them in therapeutic sessions, claiming that—like horses or dogs—these *particular* animals gain
their existence from entering this exchange. Why, then, am I legitimating
the former relations and prohibiting the latter?

Beginning with the substantial prices that horses and dogs pay for living
their lives with humans, here a liberationist is compelled to factor in
moral, political, and strategic considerations. Consider two versions of a
liberationist ideal world: The first is based on the hands-off approach.

Here, human animals live alongside nonhuman animals. Some interaction between the species might occur, but it would never be achieved through coercing animals. Pet-owner relations would probably not exist as such. People may take in injured animals for short periods, or, if they can afford the space needed, may allow animals to live and breed in an unlimited way in their homes. Cows, sheep, horses, dogs, cats, and pigs would roam freely in large areas that are fenced off from humans. They would never be killed for their flesh or hides. Nor would they be used to obtain eggs and milk: Protein substitutes would replace these, since collective moral veganism would make such replacement mandatory (and affordable). This ideal obviously involves a radical shrinking in numbers for these creatures, as there will be no financial incentive to breed them. But the ones who will exist would lead uninterrupted lives. Humans will occasionally visit these reserves (zoos would be abolished) so as to watch those animals from afar.

Here is another, less serene, liberationist ideal world: In this world, animals are never killed in order to satisfy human interests (including culinary, scientific, or recreational interests). Protein substitutes and alternative research models have been devised, activities like hunting or fishing have been outlawed, and zoos have been banished. Yet animals do live with humans in various relationships that promote some human interests. Free-roaming animals are maintained by humans so as to obtain milk and eggs. When such animals die, their flesh and hides are used. Cats, dogs, and horses are kept by humans; this does mean that they are spayed and neutered, vaccinated, and subjected to training. The animals are well kept, and some cosmetic interventions done to them today are banned.

I submit that this second ideal world is overall better for animals than the first. Many more animals would exist (millions more would exist), the lives they would lead would be qualitatively good ones and would not constitute a debasing of what having a life means—a debasement that exists when animals are perceived merely as means for producing this or that. And it is such a world that liberationists should strive to create. This does not obviously legitimize everything done to dogs or horses. Aesthetic surgery for dogs cannot be legitimated, and some modes of keeping and using horses will disappear. But this position involves embracing a quasi-paternalistic relationship with these beings, holding that doing so is beneficial to them. For a liberationist, the moral price of accepting this position is upholding the moral legitimacy of bits, harnesses, and invasive surgery. Yet for liberationists such as me, the moral price that the first world implies, although more abstract in nature, is higher: One has to, in this case, swallow the implication of a petless world, both in terms of ourselves and of these beings. And since the lives of many horses and pets are qualitatively good ones, I do not subscribe to the morally purer stance, which will make all of these disappear.

Responding to the second counter-argument requires specifying when and where the argument from non-existence can be legitimately employed. Merely bringing a being into existence is not, *ipso facto*, a benefit to it. Two additional considerations have to be brought into play before one can conclude that an entity benefits from bringing it into existence. First, the qualitative consideration: If the entity's future life is predicted to be qualitatively bad in a significant way, then bringing it into existence is not a benefit to it. The negative quality has to, of course, be significant. An obvious example is that of bringing a person into a long life of perpetual torture.[17] The second consideration is "teleological." Bringing a being into a life form, which debases the very idea of having a life, is wrong, even if the life offered is qualitatively reasonable. For example, bringing some people into the world with the sole purpose of using them as organ banks later (while providing them with a qualitatively reasonable existence) abuses what having a life means. I call this abuse "teleological," because here the problem is the distorted, projected goal for a life.

I have claimed that in the case of rodents, birds, reptiles, fish, and monkeys, there is no species-related, welfare-based justification that enables perceiving AAT as a practice that helps these beings *qua* members of a potentially extinct species. The counter-argument has granted this, yet claimed that bringing a particular member of these animals into existence for the purpose of AAT benefits the member. In response, I admit that the AAT therapist who brings a particular rodent to life for the purpose of AAT does not necessarily abuse the rodent. The life of the rodent may be comfortable, and it need not constitute a debasement of what having a life means in the same manner in which, say, factory farming abuses the lives of the animals whose lives it takes.

However, that a particular rodent does benefit from the decision to bring the rodent into existence should not change the conclusion for a liberationist. The reason for this is that when a particular AAT animal's welfare is genuinely considered, it seems overall best for the animal to be set free after being brought into existence by the therapist. And so, if the technician is truly concerned with the particular animal's welfare, the technician should hypothetically release the animal from captivity as soon as possible.

Unlike dogs or horses,—the release of whom either is not feasible in most areas (horses) or appears to compromise their welfare—mice, hamsters, and chinchillas on the whole express no particular attachment to human contact (unlike dogs) or seek their company (unlike some cats). And so, a particular, welfare-based justification from non-existence can only work if one is willing to accept the implication that the same welfare considerations, which justify bringing the particular animal into existence, would then undermine maintaining an AAT-based relationship with this particular animal, since releasing the animal is overall better for the animal.

An Exploitation-based Case for AAT?

A defender of AAT may now concede that some forms of AAT are exploitative but assert that it is morally permissible to exploit animals. This position need not be coupled with a Cartesian or a Kantian categorical denial of moral considerability to animals. The defender of AAT will here follow what appears to be the consensus in many countries: Animals are entitled to some moral considerability (and this basically means that cruelty to animals ought to be prevented). Yet nothing stands in the way of exploiting animals for all kinds of purposes, AAT included. The response to this argument ("But if it is wrong to be cruel to an entity how can it be right to exploit it"?) will be rejected by this defender of AAT by adopting a "degrees" view of moral considerability: The defender of AAT will claim that animals have some degree of moral considerability, which justifies preventing abuse of them—but not enough to prohibit exploiting them.

Yet the degrees view cannot be accepted. First, it is questionable whether it can be successfully formulated at all, though this is less important for our purposes.[18] Moreover, the morally relevant properties that generate the prohibition on cruelty—the animal's capacity to suffer as well as the animal's possession of an interest/desire not to be subjected to some actions—are shared by humans too. In the case of humans, it is partly these properties that underlie the condemnation of exploiting them. It would therefore appear mysterious why, if one is willing to admit these properties into an analysis (and condemnation) of one kind of conduct, one dismisses these very same properties when analyzing another. If, for example, one opposes cruelty to animals because their suffering is morally relevant (and not just because cruelty is reprehensible as such), one is obligated to avoid actions that create such suffering.

What this means, morally, is that when human interests appear to require animal suffering, one cannot just allow these interests to trump one's obligation to avoid creating suffering. One is morally required to seriously strive at first to devise alternatives to these conflicts of interests. Many (not all) human-animal conflicts of interests can be finessed, meaning that it is possible to meet the human need in a substantial—though sometimes not maximal—way without compromising the well being of animals. Recognizing this makes it possible to avoid a host of second-order questions regarding the relative importance of human interests as well as the plausibility (or lack of it) of mobilizing this importance in order to thwart particular animal interests.[19]

One does not have to exploit animals so as to have eggs or milk. The same applies to AAT: There are numerous effective modes of therapy that do not exploit animals; so there is no reason to institutionalize the latter. Moreover, since this essay's analysis justifies some modes of AAT— while disallowing others—if therapeutic considerations favor the use of animals, this can still be done through deploying dogs or horses. It seems strained to claim that the value of using, specifically, rodents or birds for some patients is of such additional therapeutic value (over, say, employing dogs) as to render void the desire to avoid exploitation.

Two Further Objections (and Conclusion)

The argument I have just used regarding the moral obligation to circumvent either-or conflicts of interests between humans and animals, applies also to speciesist or utilitarian objections to my general claim. "Speciesism" is a confused term and, under most of its renderings, is not opposed to liberationism.[20] In our context, a speciesist rejoinder would boil down to saying that since human interests are more important than the interests of animals, various forms of exploitation (such as the forms of AAT that rely on rodents, birds, dolphins, reptiles, and monkeys) are morally legitimate. The argument in *Two Objections* above adequately answers this objection: The question is not whose interests are more important but whether a particular conflict of interests can be avoided. Since the either-or nature of the question of some forms of AAT is a mirage, speciesism is continuous with abrogating forms of AAT that involve exploitation and can be easily replaced.

Utilitarian objections to the foregoing conclusion are similar, basically claiming that the overall good achieved in a world in which exploitative forms of AAT occur is greater than the overall good in a world that does not contain such therapeutic options. Unpacking "overall good" shows that, in the AAT context, there are three possible variants of the utilitarian claim, two of which are speciesist; the third, liberationist. The two speciesist variants of this utilitarian argument would hold that human interests are more important than animal interests. They would differ on what "more important" should mean in practice, the first variant holding that any human interest categorically trumps any animal one. The second variant maintains that some human interests trump some (though not all) animal ones.[21] The liberationist variant of a utilitarian objection, which is actually continuous with classical utilitarianism, is that human and nonhuman interests count equally; yet it may be the case that some disutility to animals, caused by exploitative forms of AAT, substantially promotes the well being of some humans in a way that makes for a better world than one in which exploitation does not occur. Responding to these objections need not invoke the complex evaluation of utilitarianism as such or the difficulties involved in weighing interests. If my previous argument is sound, considerations of an overall good only superficially imply that anyone's interests should be compromised, so all three utilitarian variants miss the mark. The therapeutic benefits to humans could be met without exploitation. Accordingly, avoiding some forms of AAT does not diminish the projected, overall good.

In conclusion: Forms of AAT that rely on horses and dogs are continuous with the welfare of these animals. Without a relationship with humans, an overwhelming number of these beings would not exist. Their lives with human beings exact a price from them. But given responsible human owners, such lives are qualitatively comfortable and safe, and they need not frustrate the social needs of these creatures. A world in which practices like AAT exist is an overall better world for these beings than one that does not include them, and this provides a broad, moral vindication of forms of AAT that rely on these beings. On the other hand, rodents, birds, monkeys, reptiles, and dolphins gain little by coercing them into AAT. Such practices are therefore exploitative. Since the human interests that are involved can be easily met without exploiting these beings, the moral conclusion is that such forms of AAT should be abolished.

Notes

1. The literature deploys a finer terminology here, distinguishing AAT from AAA (animal-assisted activities), the latter covering non-therapeutic work done with animals, which is nevertheless deemed as potentially beneficial for humans. This distinction is not pertinent to the following analysis, so I will use AAT as an umbrella term covering various modalities of therapy and assistance incorporating the use of animals.

2. Psychologically oriented AAT includes child-oriented interventions that rely on animals to achieve wide-ranging goals. These include boosting the self-esteem of insecure children: therapeutic horseback riding (hippotherapy), creating oblique communication over the child's own problems through her interaction with animals, cultivating self control and curtailing impulsive behavior in children with ADHD, enhancing empathy, responsibility, and furthering the child's capacity to nurse through creating controlled child-animal relationships. Aside from children, psychological branches of AAT also include interventions with clinically depressed individuals, with the elderly, and with incarcerated inmates in some prisons. In all, advocates of AAT claim that the ability of the animal to generate what is many times perceived as unconditional acceptance and to facilitate dialogue that is nonthreatening, their capacity to enforce on depressives or recuperating individuals a compelling "here and now," even the tactile sensations that their touch induces, turn animals into invaluable helpers in creating therapeutically meaningful interventions. Apart from allowing people to relate to themselves through projection, some psychotherapists believe that the animals tap into various unconscious drives that they embody or archetypically signify, thus creating analytically deep therapy that could not be achieved

through non-animal targeted projections. Apart from psychology, forms of AAT have been introduced in assisting the handicapped ("service animals," such as dogs for the hearing impaired, guide dogs for the blind, monkeys for quadriplegic individuals). Animals feature in programs designed to assist the mentally handicapped. They are deployed as part of new modalities of speech therapy. Animals are also relied upon to function as organic alarm systems (dogs) who can help with specific medical conditions such as epilepsy and diabetes by alerting the owner to an oncoming seizure. Specialized animal-assisted therapy programs exist for retarded individuals, for autistic people, and for patients suffering from fatal, incurable diseases. There are many available expositions of the current extent of AAT, as well as summaries of research that attempts to validate it. For some of these, see Shalev, 1996; Grammonley and Howie et al. 1997; Cusack, 1988, and Gilshtrom, 2003.

3. The terms "liberationist perspective" or "liberationist stance" are my own (drawing from Peter Singer's *Animal Liberation*). Throughout this essay such terms stipulate what I believe to be a shared consensus among various pro-animal advocates (who, needless to say, differ on many details), who would agree that the status of nonhuman animals today demands immediate reform, stemming from a prior belief that animals are not merely a resource for human usage.

4. Most surveys on AAT given above (see note 3) describe cases of manhandling and injury.

5. A different possible moral extension of considerations, which I will not attempt, relates to zoos. If keeping animals in zoos is not immoral, curtailing their movement when they are in pet centers and making life-determining decisions for them when turning them into therapeutic means will surely pass as moral too. I will avoid this direction because reversing these transitive relations does not work: A justification of animal therapy is not, *a fortiori*, a vindication of zoos, and I wish to retain the possibility that animal therapy is a justified practice, whereas the other is not.

6. My argument was made in the context of the debate among liberationists whether moral veganism or moral vegetarianism is the morally adequate response to current exploitative practice. See Zamir, 2004.

7. This claim and some of the assertions regarding horses in the next section are based on a conversation with Orit Zamir DVM.

8. A program discussed in Lannuzi and Rowan, 1991.

9. For details of this program, see Lannuzi & Rowan, 1991.

10. The surveys on AAT above usually comment on the stress and anxiety that may be involved in such programs (see, in particular on this, Lannuzi & Rowan, 1991). Animals have desires and needs, though some philosophers doubt whether these constitute interests. This subtlety does not affect my argument throughout this paper.

11. In Zamir, 2004a, I argue why the use of this argument in order to justify raising animals and killing them for their flesh is wrong. In Zamir, 2004, I suggest three restrictions on the use of this argument, which could distinguish between right and wrong applications of this argument.

12. Some philosophers would oppose this, saying that existence cannot be a benefit since this assumes a meaningless position, prior to its present existence,

in which the non-existent animal could be harmed or helped by human decisions. See Zamir, 2004, for a reply to this. Later in this essay, I summarize this reply.

13. While Cartesians seem to be more hostile than Kantians to the liberationist cause, it is interesting to note that Descartes' own position, resting as it did on the denial of animal pain, is thus conditional on an empirical belief which, when informed (and transformed) by our modern understanding regarding pain, would change the moral attitude to animals. By contrast, the Kantian indirect duties approach thoroughly repudiates the moral status of animals, and this dismissal is unconnected to the existence or non-existence of animal pain. The awareness that animals produce, and respond to, endorphins, that they respond to pain-relievers would have probably persuaded Descartes to modify his position. Kant, on the other hand, would have been unimpressed. Yet for the purposes of this essay, "Cartesians" covers all who deny that animals possess moral standing (with or without connection to pain).

14. See Zamir (2004b) "Why Animals Matter?," forthcoming in *Between the Species*.

15. Kantians and Cartesians would (rightly) charge me with an *ad hominem* reasoning here, claiming that even if AAT practitioners are likely to avoid Kantianism and Cartesianism, this predilection is no argument against these positions as being right. I admit the topical nature of my argument here and refer readers who may be interested in a more detailed response to these to Zamir, 2000b.

16. It was pointed out to me that in some dolphin-related AAT programs the dolphins are actually free and the therapeutic objectives are obtained without moving the dolphins from their natural habitat and without coercion. My remarks throughout this essay regarding dolphins do not apply to such programs.

17. This claim has no implication for discussions of euthanasia (assuming that animal- ethics discussions carry over into human-ethics). The considerations that pertain to a future life that no one yet has are different from those that are relevant to a life already possessed by a particular person. One cannot be said to benefit a future, potential life by bringing it into a projected life of perpetual fear, isolation, and pain. This does not imply that someone who already lives such a life is better off dead. The claim is also disconnected from the abortion debate, which includes its own claims regarding the relative quality of a future life. An existing zygote is a particular, potential/actual life, while we are here considering abstract, potential ones. Moreover, the negative quality of a future life of disability, of being adopted (since one's natural parents cannot responsibly function as parents), the two considerations that prompt future quality-of-a-life arguments within the abortion debate are categorically distinct from issues of projected future exploitation that are relevant here.

18. For arguments against the plausibility of a degrees view, see Rowland, 2002, Ch. 2, 3; DeGrazia, 1996, Ch. 3; Regan, 1985, Ch. 7, p. 2.

19. For discussion of the dubiousness of this move, see Zamir, 2006.

20. See Zamir, forthcoming.

21. The terminology, which has been suggested for this distinction (by Brody, 2001), is "lexical priority" of human over nonhuman interests (any human interest overmasters any animal interest) and "discounting of interests" (extremely important animal interests can take preference over negligible human interests).

References

Brody, B. A. (2001). Defending animal research: An international perspective. In E. F. Paul & J. Paul, (Eds.), *Why animal experimentation matters: The use of animals in medical research* (pp. 131–148). New Brunswick: Transaction Publishers.

Cusack, O. (1988). *Pets and mental health*, NY: Haworth Press.

DeGrazia, D. (1996). *Taking animals seriously: Mental life and moral status*, NY: Cambridge University Press.

Gilshtrom, R. (2003). *Special pets for special needs population*. Israel: Ach (Hebrew).

Grammonley, J., Howie, A. R., Kirwin, S., Zapf, S., Frye, J., Freeman, G., Stuart-Lannuzi, D. & Rowan, A. N. (1991). Ethical issues in animal-assisted therapy programs, *Anthrozoös*, 4 (3), 154–163.

Preziosi, R. J. (1997). For your consideration: A pet-assisted therapist facilitator code of ethics, *The Latham Letter*, Spring, pp. 5–6.

Rowland, M. (2002). *Animals like us*, London: Verso.

Regan, T. (1985). *The case for animals rights*, Berkeley: University of California Press.

Shalev, A. (1996). *The furry healer: Pets as a therapeutic means: Theory, research and practice*, Tel-Aviv: Tcherikover Publishers (Hebrew).

Zamir, T. (2004). Veganism, *Journal of Social Philosophy*, September, 35 (3), 367–379.

Zamir, T. (2004a, June). Killing for pleasure, *Between the Species* (web-journal).

Zamir, T. (2004b). Why animals matter? *Between the Species* (web-journal).

Zamir, T. (2006). Killing for knowledge, *Journal of Applied Philosophy*.

Zamir, T. (forthcoming). *Is speciesism opposed to liberationism?*

Index

About the Author

Donald Altschiller is a librarian at Mugar Memorial Library at Boston University, Boston, MA. He has written several reference books, including ABC-CLIO's *Hate Crimes: A Reference Handbook*. He has also contributed articles to many encyclopedias, is a long-time reviewer for *Library Journal* and *Choice*, and has served on the editorial board of *Reference Books Bulletin*.